DADHOOD UNPLUGGED

THE ESSENTIAL GUIDE FOR
FIRST-TIME DADS

Handy Tips to Build a Bond with Your Baby,
Support Your Partner Actively, Reduce Emotional Anxiety
and Achieve Work-Life Harmony

akin olunloyo

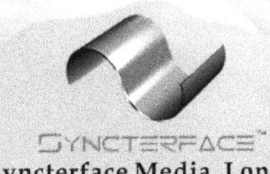

Syncterface Media, London
www.syncterfacemedia.com

Copyright © 2025 by akin olunloyo

Published in the United Kingdom by Syncterface Media Ltd. | www.syncterfacemedia.com

Cover design by Simply Sumfink
Interior design by Hart Vybes inc
Illustrations courtesy of the author

All rights reserved. No part of this book may be reproduced by any mechanical, photographic, or electronic process, or in the form of a phonographic recording; nor may it be stored in a retrieval system, transmitted, or otherwise be copied for public or private use—other than for "fair use" as brief quotations embodied in articles and reviews - without prior written permission of the publisher.

The author of this book does not dispense medical advice or prescribe the use of any technique as a form of treatment for physical, emotional, or medical problems. The intent of the author is only to offer information of a general nature to help you in your quest to be the best dad you can be. In the event you use any of the information in this book for yourself, the author and the publisher assume no responsibility for your actions.

Paperback ISBN: 978-1-912896-97-4
eBook ISBN: 978-1-912896-98-1
Audiobook ISBN: 978-1-912896-99-8

*To my lovely angels,
Oyindamola and Oluwatishe,
for doing what they do best:
Showering their dad with love.*

DADHOOD
UNPLUGGED
redefining fatherhood

Contents

Foreword ix

The Intro xi

Dadhood Unplugged   1
Redefining Fatherhood: The Dadhood Mindset 1
Assembling Your Dream Team: Friends, Family, and Beyond 4
No One-Size-Fits-All 8

The Dynamic Duo   11
Mastering the Art of Communication 11
Enhancing Your Relationship 13
Sparking Passion and Romance During Pregnancy 16

The Expectant Dad   19
And So the Journey Begins 19
Maternity Planning: Expenses, Resources and Lifelines 22
Budgeting for Baby Essentials 27

The Nine-Month Adventure   33
Journeying Through Trimesters 33
Navigating the Twists and Turns Together 35

The Big Push   43
The Birth Plan: Your Delivery Blueprint 43
Embracing Your Birth Duties 45
The Labour Ward: Tips and Need-to-Knows 46
Labour Unveiled 47
Baby's First Hello 49

Baby Bootcamp ~ Phase I   53
Embrace the Unpredictability 53
The Round-the-Clock Buffet 54
Sleep,... or the Lack Thereof 59

Baby Bootcamp ~ Phase II   63
Diapering 101: Handling the Mess with Ease 63
Bathing and Hygiene: Keeping Baby Clean 67
Soothing Techniques: Calming a Fussy Baby 71

The Fourth Trimester   75
Post-Childbirth Reality Check 75
Balancing Support and Personal Well-being 78

Keeping the Romance Alive 82

The Bonding — 85
Kangaroo Care Moments 85
Babywearing 87
Stimulating Your Baby's Development 89
Creative Bonding Activities 90
Baby Cues: The Must Learn Language 92
The Key is in the Two P's 94
Cherish Every Moment 95

Sharing the Dad Love — 97

Health and Happiness — 99
Understanding Your Baby's Vital Signs 99
Common Health Issues 100
Your Baby's Immunity and Well-Being 103
First Aid Basics for First-Time Dads 105
Your Well-Being: Emotional, Physical and Mental 108

Safe and Secure — 111
Creating a Safe Haven 111
Sweet Dreams, Safe Slumbers 114
Avoiding Food Fiascos 115
Splash and Secure 117
Baby-Safe Travels 118
In a Nutshell 120

Baby's Greatest Hits — 121
Zero to Three Months: Survival Mode 121
Three to Six Months: The Wiggle Phase 122
Four to Six Months: The Soundtrack of Laughter 123
Six to Nine Months: The Mobile Era 124
Six to Twelve Months: The Culinary Adventures 125
Nine to Twelve Months: Talking and Walking 127
Capturing Special Moments 129

Growing Your Baby's Wealth — 133
Set Goals and Priorities 133
Build an Emergency Fund 134
Start a Savings Account 135
Investing for Your Child's Future 137
Education Savings Plans 139

Future-Proofing Your Little One — 143

Maximising Tax Benefits 143
　　Life Insurance 145
　　Creating a Will 147
　　Teaching Financial Literacy 148
　　Final Nuggets 149

Mastering the Juggle   151
　　Set Priorities 151
　　Become a Scheduling Ninja 153
　　Roll with the Punches 154
　　Protect Your Personal Time 155
　　Let Go of the Pressure 157
　　Reflect and Adjust 158
　　Parental Leave: The Fears, the Joys and the Realities 159
　　In Conclusion 163

Faith-Filled Dadhood   165
　　A New Dimension 165
　　Words of Wisdom 170

Laughing Through Dadhood   171
　　A Touch of Magic 171
　　The Sweet Melody of Laughter 175

Must-Haves for New Dads   177
　　The Essential Gear Toolkit 177
　　The Tech Toolkit 180
　　The "Must-Reads" Toolkit 182
　　The "Online Resources" Toolkit 183
　　The Emotional Toolkit 185
　　Final Thoughts 187

The Outro   189

Acknowledgements   193

About Akin   196

Glossary   198

References   212

Keep the Dadhood Spirit Alive   219

Dadhood is...

"...the dynamic blend of nurturing, guidance, and partnership."

~ akin.o ~

Foreword

What you hold in your hand is, without a doubt, a resource that will be invaluable at differing times of your journey of being a dad, however long or short that may be.

What Akin has been able to pull together is more than just an academic piece of work. This is something that is completely him. It is Akin's passion and journey as a friend, husband, father and most of all, a dad. A generous combination of an unshakeable belief in God, strength, awareness, kindness, perception, diligence and doggedness has been woven into the words on the pages of this book for when the reader will need them most.

If I look back to when I first became a dad, a memory that simultaneously warms my heart and brings tears of gratitude to my eyes, this book would have been invaluable back then. The information, humour, and principles Akin so eloquently presents in this book make it a poor candidate to read cover to cover, put on your shelf, and forget. Rather you will likely pick it up when times are good and otherwise, when going on holiday or on the way to a busy day at the office. Just like a wise, good and trusted friend, it will be there when you need it most.

I have absolutely no doubt that what you are about to read will bless you and I wholly commend it to you. Refer to it when you need it, and refer to it when you don't. When you need to smile, underline the jokes and the funny parts for the truths they hide will stay with you forever and when you need some honest, well-meaning advice that reassures you that you are not the only one.

Being a father is a God-given privilege, but being a dad is a choice.

You will do great!

- BAJO AKISANYA
Pastor | Youth & Young Adult Minister | Empowerment Coach | Voice Actor
Jesus House for All Nations, London

The Intro
Welcome to Dadhood

Welcome to "The Essential Guide for First-Time Dads", your ultimate sidekick, packed with real talk, helpful advice, and a healthy dose of humour. This guide is here to help you navigate the sometimes chaotic, often hilarious, and always rewarding wild ride of being a father. So, grab a snack, settle in, and let's dive into the wonderful world of modern-day fatherhood, or what I simply call dadhood.

When I first held my daughter in my arms, I realised I was holding the most delicate, beautiful, and maybe terrifying thing I had ever encountered. She looked up at me with eyes full of love and wonder, and I thought, "Well, here we go. Welcome to the world of full-on responsibility." I had spent a few months preparing for this moment, reading books and articles. Yet, there I was, feeling like someone who had just been handed the keys to a spaceship with no idea how to fly it. Clueless! *(Interestingly, I had almost the same feeling when I held my second daughter nearly four years later)* Maybe, just like me, you're feeling a cocktail of emotions; excitement, fear, joy and sheer panic. Let me assure you, it's perfectly normal.

Being a dad today is a whole different ballgame. Gone are the days when dads were just the breadwinners, disciplinarians or the guys who fix things around the house. Now, we're expected to be emotionally tuned in, ready to change a diaper at a moment's notice and the master of bedtime storytelling. Research shows that engaged dads can make a world of difference in a child's life. We're talking about better emotional health, stronger academic performance, and even improved social skills. Plus, you get the added bonus of building a strong bond with your child and creating memories that will last a lifetime. Who knew that being a dad could be so rewarding?

So, what makes this book different from the others? For starters, it's not just about how to change a diaper or burp a baby. Although, don't worry, I've got you covered there too. This book takes a holistic approach. It's about keeping your relationship strong and maintaining a balanced work-life routine. It's about emotional well-being and growing not just as a dad but as a partner and an individual. So, even though these pages are intended to prepare you for the little one to come, they will also make you a better person.

And who is this book for? Whether you're a first-time dad, a curious partner, or anyone looking for a relatable and informative guide on dadhood, this book is for you. It doesn't matter where you live, whether in the United Kingdom, across the pond, or anywhere else; you'll find the content relevant and engaging. This book is inclusive and aims to support anyone stepping into the role of a dad.

On the pages of this guide, we'll talk about preparing for dadhood, supporting your partner, what to expect during pregnancy, navigating the newborn phase, baby bonding, health and safety, and even the elusive work-life balance. There'll also be some valuable tips on how to keep your relationship alive, manage emotional anxiety, understand common health concerns and help out with your little one's financial future. We'll cover everything from the practical to the emotional, with a few dad jokes thrown in for good measure. My prayer is that by the end of this book, you'll find everything you need to feel confident and prepared for the dadhood journey ahead.

And just in case you're wondering why I've decided to put this guide together. Well, that's simple. Apart from being a father of two daughters who has had his fair share of reading bedtime stories, changing countless diapers and navigating the delicate balance of work and family life, I have also had the opportunity to talk to several new dads. The common theme seems to be that it would be great if they had an easy guide to shed some light on this dadhood thing. Well, it's all here, ready for you to explore and ensure you don't drown in the details.

As someone who has been there, I know how much it means to have someone in your corner as a first-time dad. So, I invite you to jump on the dadhood train and embrace this incredible adventure filled with highs and lows, challenges and triumphs. I assure you that your life will be transformed in ways you never imagined. Remember, millions of dads have walked this path before you. You're not alone. Together, we'll navigate your new chapter. Welcome to dadhood - it's going to be a blast!

Dadhood is...

"...the art of being present, engaged, and committed to raising happy, well-rounded, and respectful kids while also prioritising open communication, promoting equality, and striving to create a loving environment for the family."

~ akin.o ~

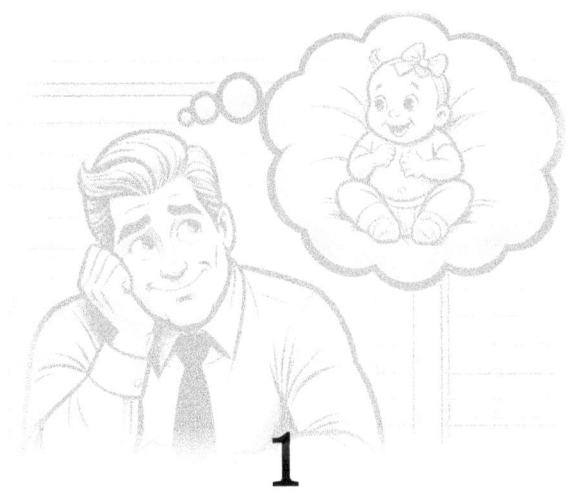

1

Dadhood Unplugged
Let the Fun Begin

There's a moment that never leaves you as an expectant dad. It might hit you during a midnight snack raid or as you fumble with the cot assembly in the wee hours of the morning. For me, it was while watching my wife's belly move as our daughter performed what seemed like a gymnastics routine inside her. Suddenly, the reality of becoming a dad was more vivid than ever. It was both exhilarating and terrifying. Not as if I didn't know, but let's say it dawned on me that it wasn't just about assembling a cot at an odd hour; it was about preparing myself to become the kind of father who could meet both the needs of my child and the new era expectations of dadhood.

Redefining Fatherhood: The Dadhood Mindset

Today's fathers are redefining what it means to be a dad. We're dismantling the old stereotypes of distant breadwinners and disciplinarians and embracing roles that include emotional involvement, active caregiving, and true partnership in parenting. In the past, fathers were often seen as the strong, silent type, expected to focus on providing while mothers managed the home. However, changing societal attitudes are reshaping these expectations. Research shows that children whose dads engage in their emotional and developmental growth tend to flourish mentally, socially and even academically. So, whether you're a dad who stays home or one who works long hours, your involvement is vital.

Emotional Intelligence

Emotional intelligence is now as crucial as financial acumen. Understanding and responding to your child's emotions are as important as knowing how to change a diaper. Don't get me wrong, I'm not saying you should disregard the old ways of fatherhood. But a blend of old-school wisdom and new-age sensitivity will go a long way to making your child well-rounded. Balancing the traditional roles with modern expectations may involve a bit of juggling, but it's worth it. You're not just preparing to be a dad; you're preparing to be a superhero in your child's eyes.

Tackling Emotions

As a first-time dad, you might experience a rollercoaster of emotions, from being thrilled at the thought of meeting your little one to being overwhelmed by the responsibility, from sheer joy to overwhelming anxiety; the spectrum of emotions is vast and ever-changing. Well, the good news is, it's perfectly normal. You're not alone in wondering whether you'll be a good dad or how you'll manage sleepless nights and diaper changes. These worries are a natural part of your journey into dadhood. The trick is to acknowledge and embrace these feelings and not brush them under the rug. During pregnancy, take time to self-reflect. Take time to understand how you're feeling and why. This self-awareness will help you navigate the emotional stages of dadhood, from anticipating your baby's arrival to the reality of holding them for the first time. Remember, it's okay to feel some form of anxiety and self-doubt. They're signals that you care deeply about doing a good job. So, take a deep breath and know that you're doing great.

Building Dad Confidence

Then there's the confidence issue. Building confidence in your ability to father begins with education. The more you know, the more prepared you'll feel. You can start by diving into some recommended reading for expectant dads. There are plenty of books out there that offer insights and practical advice. You could also look at online courses, as they can be a great resource when it comes to providing the basics of dadhood in a digestible format. And don't forget about prenatal classes. Attending these with your partner can offer a wealth of information and help you feel more prepared. Remember, the more you know, the more confident you'll be in your role as a dad. It's like preparing for a marathon - you train, you read up on techniques, and you practice. It's all about building a solid foundation.

Mastering the Art of Imperfection

Don't take the importance of setting practical, personal expectations for granted, as this can ease the transition into dadhood. It's easy to fall into the trap of perfectionism, wanting to be the perfect dad who never makes a mistake. But newborns are unpredictable, and no amount of planning can account for every scenario. So, dads who adapt and learn on the fly often fare best. Try to find a balance between planning and improvisation, and understand that though your best may vary from day to day, it's okay. By setting realistic expectations, you're setting yourself up for success. Flexibility is your ally. Embrace the unpredictability of this new phase and the unique challenges it brings. It's a journey, not a destination.

Crafting the Ultimate Dad Vision
Finally, it's time to create your vision for dadhood. Take a moment to define your core values and priorities. What kind of dad do you aspire to be? Do you want to be the dad who's at every soccer game or the one who's known for bedtime stories and silly voices? Do you want to build a relationship with your child that's based on trust, openness, and love? Envision your relationship with your child and the memories you want to create. Paint a picture in your mind of the dad-child relationship you hope to cultivate. This picture will guide you through the ups and downs and remind you of what truly matters. So, take a step back, reflect, and embrace the dad you're becoming. Remember, it's not just about being present; it's about being intentional with your time and efforts. Start building this vision now, adjusting as you learn and grow alongside your child. Trust me, it's going to be an incredible adventure.

Assembling Your Dream Team: Friends, Family, and Beyond

Once again, it's the wee hours of the morning, and you're wide awake, cradling a baby who seems to have swapped sleep for a newfound fascination with the ceiling fan. Your partner is snoring softly, catching those precious and well-deserved z's, and you're wondering if your definition of sleep will ever be the same again. What you wouldn't give for a helping hand.

It Takes a Village
"It takes a village to raise a child" is a common saying, and it's very true. When you find yourself in the midst of dadhood, you'll realise just how valuable that village is. Picture it as a

relay race. Sure, you're running the track, but you've got a team cheering you on, ready to hand you a water bottle or take the baton when you need a breather. As you step into this new role, the importance of knowing you have a tribe you can rely on cannot be overstated. It's like assembling your own personal team of superheroes, each with a unique power.

Your support squad isn't just there to coo over the little one while you catch a nap - although that is a definite perk. They provide the emotional buoyancy needed to stay afloat amidst the waves of sleepless nights and endless diaper changes. They offer a shoulder to lean on, especially in the tough times. They share your joys and frustrations. They can be a sounding board and, sometimes, a much-needed reality check. One thing to remember is that a robust support system not only provides a helping hand but also a reassuring presence that says, "You're not in this alone."

Rallying the Tribe

Identifying your potential support network is your first step. Think of the people who have always been there for you and your partner, the ones you can rely on without hesitation. Make a list of people you trust - family members, close friends, and trustworthy colleagues who are parents themselves. Consider those who are ever ready to lend an ear or offer advice, those who have always been there for you.

But don't stop there - reach out to them. Think about how to initiate supportive conversations. A simple, "Hey, I might need some help when the baby arrives. Can I count on you?" goes a long way. More often than not, people are eager to lend a hand; they just need a little nudge. Strategies for reaching out include being open about your needs and expressing gratitude for their support. Remember, asking for help isn't a sign of weakness; it's a testament to your dedication as a parent.

The Power of Support Groups

This might not be every first-time dad's cup of tea, but joining a dad group you can relate with could be a game-changer. These groups, whether local meetups or online communities, offer a sense of kinship and understanding that's hard to find elsewhere.

- Local support groups provide face-to-face interaction and a chance to share stories and advice over a hot chocolate. They're like a secret club where everyone understands what you're going through, a relaxed, judgement-free zone where you can talk about the funny, the frustrating, and the downright bizarre aspects of dadhood, a space where you can simply connect with other dads who get it. Whether you're seeking advice on handling sleepless nights, figuring out the best diaper brands, or just wanting to chat about your latest dad win, these groups provide a great mix of camaraderie and practical support. Plus, they can be a fantastic way to build friendships that extend beyond the parenting realm.

Finding a support group that fits your schedule and vibe might take some trial and error, and opening up to strangers can be daunting at first. But once you find the right group, the pros often far outweigh the cons, providing invaluable support on your dadhood journey.

- Online communities and social media groups expand your reach, connecting you with dads from all walks of life and creating a vibrant hub of shared experiences, advice, and fellowship. They're like dependable digital lifelines, especially when you're feeling isolated. Whether you're looking for tips on managing sleepless nights, recommendations for the best baby gear, or just want to connect with other dads who get it, these groups offer a wealth of knowledge and support. They're also accessible anytime, anywhere. The convenience of connecting from home, often in your pyjamas with a cuppa in your hand, is hard to beat. From Facebook groups to specialised forums, these online communities provide a sense of kinship and connection that can make the journey of dadhood a little less daunting and a lot more enjoyable.

While online communities offer valuable resources and support, they come with downsides like privacy risks and the overwhelming volume of information. To stay safe, use pseudonyms, limit profile information, and avoid sharing personal details, especially about your children. Also, navigating conflicting advice can be challenging, and the lack of face-to-face interaction may hinder personal connections. But, despite these issues, thoughtful participation in online groups can be a fantastic resource for navigating dadhood.

In this ever-connected world, finding a community can be a lifeline for dads seeking support and camaraderie. It's about finding a space where you can be yourself, share your triumphs and struggles, and learn from others walking a similar path. Remember, parenting is a shared journey; there's strength in numbers. Whether you're looking for advice, a laugh, or just a place to vent, these communities offer a wealth of possibilities.

Embracing Professional Help
Sometimes, despite our best efforts, we might find ourselves needing a bit more support. This is where professional help steps in. There's no shame in seeking it; in fact, it shows a proactive approach to parenting. Whether it's seeking advice from a doctor regarding your baby's health, consulting a financial advisor to plan for your child's future, or talking to a therapist or counsellor for emotional support, these professionals offer valuable expertise that can make your parenting journey smoother. It's a chance to work through any anxieties or concerns you might have, guided by someone

who's trained to help. Parenting workshops and seminars also provide valuable insights and strategies, equipping you with the tools needed to thrive as a new dad. Embracing professional support can strengthen your confidence and enhance your ability to support your partner and child. So, take advantage of the resources available, and don't hesitate to lean on the pros – they're a big part of your dream team!

Teamwork Makes the Dream Work
Building a support team is about creating a circle of trust and care that extends beyond your immediate family. It's about finding those who uplift you, who know the ups and downs of parenthood, and who you can depend on through the good times and bad. It's about recognising the strength of community and the power of shared experiences. As you navigate dadhood, lean on your crew. Allow them to celebrate the milestones with you and help carry the load when it feels too heavy. Remember, you're not in this alone. You've got a whole team cheering you on, ready to support you every step of the way. As you continue on this path, take comfort in knowing that your village is there, ready to help you raise your child with care, wisdom, and so much love. And if you just happen to be a person of faith, remember there's a Special Someone who is always there, always ready to lend a helping hand whenever you need one.

No One-Size-Fits-All

Today, dads are stepping up in new and exciting ways, breaking the moulds of old and stepping into roles that go beyond traditional expectations. Midnight feeds, changing nappies, having heart-to-heart chats, or simply being a steady presence are now dadhood norms. Today's dads understand that they don't have to navigate dadhood alone and that leaning on a trustworthy support network makes them stronger and better. Dadhood isn't about having all the answers or being perfect; it's about being present. It's about showing up, learning on the fly, embracing the highs and lows, and sometimes just winging it with a lot of love and patience. If there's one thing I know, it's this: There's no one-size-fits-all approach to being a dad. So, embrace the season, laugh at the mishaps, celebrate the little victories, and cherish every perfectly imperfect moment. Remember, being a dad is one of the most rewarding adventures, so don't be afraid to make a difference in your own unique way!

"Caregiving, role modelling, sharing and
Embracing the joys and challenges of parenting;
That's Dadhood!

Remember,
In every joy, in every tear,
A real dad is always there."

~ akin.o ~

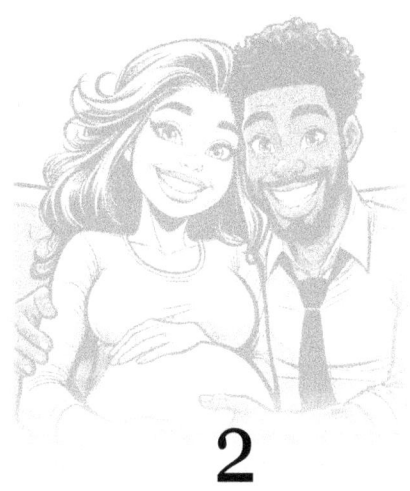

2

The Dynamic Duo
Just the Two of Us

Being a first-time parent is a thrilling adventure, but it's also a team sport, and communication with your partner on all levels is the lifeline that will keep you both anchored. This chapter is all about making sure you and your partner are in sync, like a dynamic duo ready to face whatever parenthood throws your way.

Mastering the Art of Communication

Communication is a funny thing. We often think we're great at it until we're faced with a partner who just wants us to listen without offering a solution or a fix. Enter the art of empathetic listening.

Empathetic Listening
This is where you turn off the problem-solving brain and genuinely tune in to what your partner is saying. Empathetic listening is like having a superpower that transforms your

conversations from mundane exchanges into meaningful dialogues. By practising active listening techniques - like giving your full attention, making eye contact, and nodding along - you create a space where your partner feels heard and understood. Reflecting back what you hear is a game-changer. It shows that you're not just hearing words but absorbing the emotions behind them. It's amazing what a little empathy can do to deepen your connection.

Decoding Emotional Cues

But how can you tell when your partner needs you to listen? Recognising emotional cues is vital. Imagine your partner's emotions are like a weather report. Sunny smiles mean all is well, while stormy expressions might indicate trouble brewing. Understanding non-verbal communication is essential here. A sigh could mean they're feeling overwhelmed, while crossed arms might signal discomfort or frustration. Identifying these stress indicators allows you to respond with the appropriate level of support. Maybe it's a reassuring hug or a simple "I'm here for you." By being attuned to these cues, you create a supportive atmosphere where your partner feels safe to express themselves.

The Right Words

When it comes to expressing support, words matter. Using "I" statements instead of "you" can make a world of difference in how your message is received. Saying "I feel worried when you're stressed" instead of "You're always stressed" can prevent defensiveness and foster understanding. Validating your partner's emotions is another powerful tool. Acknowledging their feelings with phrases like "That sounds really tough" or "I can see why you'd feel that way" can make them feel valued and appreciated. Even during disagreements, maintaining supportive communication is essential. It's all about understanding each other's perspectives and finding common ground.

Delicate Discussions

Navigating difficult conversations requires sensitivity and care. It's like walking through a field of daisies, trying not to crush any delicate blooms. Setting a calm and private time for these discussions is crucial. You don't want to dive into a heavy topic when you're both exhausted or distracted. Agreeing on shared goals and compromises can help you reach a resolution without conflict. Remember, you're a team, not adversaries. The aim is to work together towards a solution that strengthens your relationship.

Never forget that your relationship with your partner is the foundation upon which your parenting adventure is built. By improving your communication skills, you're not only enhancing your relationship but also setting a positive example for your little one(s). Remember, you're in this together, and with a bit of compassion and understanding, you'll be ready to face any challenge that comes your way.

Enhancing Your Relationship

You and your partner are sitting on the couch, all hugged up, and there is a rare moment of warm quiet stretching between you. You look into each other's eyes and realise that, amidst the chaos of work, life and pregnancy, you've taken one crucial thing for granted - connecting with each other. This is where understanding love languages comes into play. Introduced by Gary Chapman, the concept of love languages is simple yet profound. It's about understanding how we give and receive love, which can totally transform relationships.

The Fantastic Five
Knowing your partner's love language is like having the secret recipe to their happiness. That said, pregnancy has a funny way of turning everything upside down, even changing the dynamics of love languages. Just when you thought you had

your partner's love language(s) in the bag, she flipped it. That is why adapting is key. So, first, figure out your partner's primary love language – the one that speaks louder than the others. And once you're up-to-date, it's time to start sprinkling a little love magic into your daily routine.

- **Words of Affirmation.** If this is your partner's love language, try to find ways to express love, appreciation, and affection through verbal compliments, encouraging words, and supportive affirmations. A simple "You're doing an amazing job" or "I'm so proud of you" can make all the difference. These little confidence boosts can reassure and uplift your partner, showing them you're in this together. Whether it's complimenting their strength or expressing your love and appreciation, your words can be a comforting anchor through all the ups and downs. Remember, every kind word adds to a stronger, more connected time together.

- **Acts of Service.** If it's this one, then it's all about showing love through helpful actions. Tackling the mountain of laundry, cooking up your partner's favourite meal, doing the dishes, or simply making her a cuppa are things that easily come to mind. These gestures might seem small, but they speak volumes about your love and support. By taking care of these little tasks, you're letting your partner know you're in this together, making their life a bit easier, and showing them that you've got their back every step of the way. It's all about being a thoughtful, hands-on partner during this exciting journey.

- **Receiving Gifts.** Pregnancy is a special time, so if this is your partner's love language, here's your chance to add a magic touch. Remember, it's not really about flashy or expensive presents – it's the thought that counts. Surprise your partner with a box of her most cherished chocolates, a bouquet of her favourite flowers, or a heartfelt letter. Or you could consider thoughtful tokens of appreciation such as a handmade card or even a playlist of her favourite songs. These small, meaningful gifts show that you're thinking of her and want to make her feel special. It's all about finding little ways to brighten her day and reminding her that you're in this together. A well-timed gift can be a lovely gesture to lift her spirits and show your love and appreciation.

- **Quality Time.** If your partner craves undivided attention, I personally believe this is one of the best ways to show your love and support. It's all about being fully present and sharing meaningful moments together. Whether it's binge-watching your favourite series, planning a surprise date night with no distractions, or just having a heartfelt chat, these moments of togetherness will surely strengthen your bond. Taking time to listen, laugh, and connect with your partner can make her feel special and loved. It's about creating those precious memories and showing that you're walking side by side, enjoying every step along the way.

- **Physical Touch.** Now, this can be incredibly comforting and reassuring for your partner during pregnancy if she's a physical touch lover. Simple gestures like a kiss on the forehead, holding hands, gentle back rubs, or cuddling on the couch can help her feel loved and supported. These touches provide not only physical comfort but also create an emotional connection, showing that you're there for her through every kick, craving, and mood swing. A warm hug or a soft touch on the shoulder can make all the difference in making her feel cherished and cared for. It's all about being present and showing your love through those small, meaningful touches.

Incorporating love languages into your relationship is a bit like adding seasoning to a dish - it enhances the flavour and brings out the best in each other. It's about recognising that love isn't a one-size-fits-all thing, and by speaking each other's language, you're creating a deeper, more fulfilling connection. This isn't just about getting through the day-to-day; it's about flourishing together, even amidst the challenges of pregnancy. Understanding and applying love languages can transform your relationship into something truly special, where love is expressed in ways that genuinely resonate with both you and your partner.

Creating a Love Symphony
Balancing love languages with personal needs is like walking on a tightrope. It's crucial to find harmony between meeting your partner's needs and expressing your own love language. This is where honest communication comes into play. Share your needs and preferences openly. Let your partner know what makes you feel loved and appreciated, and encourage them to do the same. It's about creating a reciprocal flow of love where both partners feel valued. Encourage acts of love that resonate with both of you. Perhaps you both enjoy watching romantic movies or cooking together. These shared activities can be a fusion of love languages, enhancing your connection. Remember, even though pregnancy may shift your priorities, it doesn't have to dampen your ability to express love.

Sparking Passion and Romance During Pregnancy

Pregnancy is a time of incredible transformation, not just for your partner but for your relationship as well. As her body changes, so might her comfort levels and desires. Sparking passion during this time can be a wonderful way to keep the romance alive. It's all about finding those little moments to show love and affection, even when life gets a bit hectic. Think of it as adding an extra spark to your relationship's glow.

Physical Intimacy
Let's face it, intimacy can be a bit of a puzzle when you're

navigating a body that's growing a whole person. Finding comfortable positions for intimacy becomes crucial, and creativity is your new best friend. Think of it as a fun challenge rather than a chore. Whether it's switching up locations or exploring different ways to be close, the key is to maintain a sense of humour and openness. Embrace non-sexual forms of closeness too. Simple acts like holding hands or cuddling on the couch can be just as rewarding and help maintain that connection.

Emotional Intimacy

Beyond the physical, pregnancy is a prime time to nurture emotional intimacy. Sharing your hopes and fears about parenthood can be incredibly bonding. Once again, it's about opening up those lines of communication and being vulnerable with each other. Engage in joint activities or hobbies, whether that's a leisurely walk in the park or something more structured like doing a jigsaw puzzle. These shared experiences create memories and strengthen your bond. Emotional intimacy is the glue that holds you together, especially when the going gets tough.

Creating Together Moments

With a baby on the way, it's easy to get caught up in the frenzy of life and forget about the romance. But, maintaining a strong connection is essential. Plan a date night. It doesn't have to be extravagant; sometimes, a picnic in the backyard or a night under the stars is all it takes. Write letters or notes to each other. Yes, it might sound old-fashioned, but there's something magical about putting pen to paper. Engage in couple's relaxation sessions to unwind and reconnect. These moments of togetherness are precious, so make them count.

Love Reassured

Of course, with all these changes, it's natural to have concerns or apprehensions about intimacy. Addressing these openly is very important. Honest conversations about changing desires can be a relief. It's about creating a space where both of you feel safe to express your needs and concerns. Reassure each other of your love and attraction. A simple "I love you" or "You're beautiful" can work wonders. Remember, pregnancy is a temporary phase, and the love you share is the constant that will see you through.

Remember that intimacy is more than just the physical. It's about connection, trust, and understanding. Nurture these aspects, and you'll find that the bond you share with your partner will grow stronger each day.

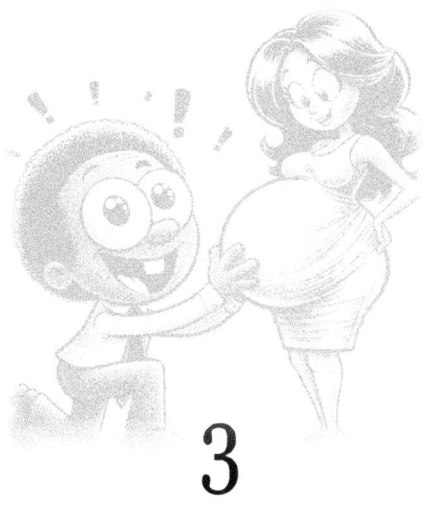

3

The Expectant Dad
Plans, Lifelines and Budgets

Now, we all know your partner is doing most of the heavy lifting, but never underestimate the part you play. From the elation of the first positive test to the late-night snack runs, your journey will be filled with unique moments and surprises. So, buckle up, dad-to-be, because this is where the magic happens, and trust me, you're in for the experience of a lifetime.

And So the Journey Begins

Welcome to the world of antenatal (prenatal) appointments. The first is often a mixed bag of emotions. It's like embarking on a tour of the exciting unknown. You and your partner walk in, heart racing with excitement and a touch of nerves, ready to take on the adventure together. As the midwife welcomes you both with a warm smile, you feel like you've just met your friendly tour guide. But you're still wondering what on earth this appointment actually entails. Don't worry, you're not alone.

Entering the Unknown

The first visit is more like a get-to-know meet and greet. The midwife will gather all the baseline information about your partner's health and also do things like confirm the pregnancy and estimate the due date. You might also get to experience that magical moment when you hear your baby's tiny heartbeat for the first time. It's like the ultimate soundtrack to this adventure. I'd advise taking a box of tissues along because there's a high possibility that the joy tears will flow. Also, we all know that medical jargon can sometimes feel like a foreign language, so don't hesitate to ask questions for clarification. Your healthcare professional is a pro at this stuff, and I'm sure they'll willingly provide the answers you need. By the end of this appointment, you'll both be buzzing with excitement, ready for the next chapter in this amazing journey.

What to Expect Next

After the first one, antenatal (prenatal) appointments become a regular gig. Each is an opportunity to check your baby's growth and development as well as your partner's health, ensuring everything is on track. They might feel like routine check-ups, but each visit is a step closer to meeting your little one. Here's a quick rundown of what you might encounter:

- **Ultrasounds.** These are the big guns of antenatal (prenatal) care and perhaps the most anticipated appointments, where you get the first glimpse of your little one. Watching your baby wiggle around on the screen is like watching the best movie ever - directed by nature, starring your kid. Ultrasounds are crucial in monitoring your baby's development.

- **Blood Tests.** Okay, these might not be as glamorous, but they provide essential information about your partner's health and the baby's well-being. From checking blood types and iron levels to screening for gestational diabetes, these tests are vital in ensuring a healthy pregnancy.

- **Measurements.** Here's where the healthcare professional breaks out the measuring tape to check the size of your partner's belly and ensure your baby's growing at a healthy rate and everything is on track. It's one of those reassuring moments where you get a tangible sense of your baby's progress. Remember, each centimetre brings you one step closer to meeting your little one!

Antenatal (prenatal) appointments provide invaluable insights, helping you prepare for the journey ahead with confidence.

More Than a Spectator

It's easy to feel like a sidekick during these appointments, but your role is crucial.

- **During Appointments.** It's not just about being physically present; it's about showing up as an involved partner and being there for your loved one. Be supportive, ask questions, take notes, and show interest. Whether it's holding your partner's hand during an uncomfortable test or just being there to hear the results, your presence matters. Participating in these visits is your golden ticket to understanding pregnancy from a front-row seat.

- **After Appointments.** Your role doesn't end once the appointment is over. After visits, reflecting on the information together can help both of you feel more grounded. Take some time to discuss new insights or advice from your healthcare professional and plan your next steps. Maybe it's a change in diet or a new exercise routine. Whatever it is, make it a team effort. By supporting your partner post-appointment, you're reinforcing the bond that will carry you through the coming months.

According to *HealthyChildren.org*, your involvement in these early stages significantly impacts both the pregnancy and your relationship with your partner. So, be present. Who knows, you might just find yourself becoming the "pregnancy whisperer," translating medical jargon into plain English. Remember, your presence is a reminder that you're both in this together, ready to embrace the challenges and joys of pregnancy with open arms.

Let the Countdown Begin
As the due date approaches, things will start to get real. Packing the hospital bag, installing the car seat, and setting up the cot (crib) will become your new hobbies. Embrace it. There will be highs and lows. One moment, you'll be over the moon, and the next, you'll be fretting over test results or pregnancy symptoms. It's normal to feel a bit overwhelmed. Talk to your partner, share your worries, and remember you're in this together. Antenatal (prenatal) appointments are just the beginning, but they're an essential part of the adventure. So, stay involved and stay positive. Soon enough, you'll be holding your baby in your arms, and all these appointments will feel like a blur.

Maternity Planning: Expenses, Resources and Lifelines

Now that you've got that dad-to-be glow, let's talk about the not-so-glamorous side of expecting a baby - expenses. Though dreaming about cute baby clothes and adorable nurseries may make you feel giddy with delight and excitement, the reality is you must first tackle the numbers. So, let me try to make navigating these expenses a bit more straightforward.

Healthcare Costs in the UK
So, what's the actual cost of maternity care? Well, that would depend on where you're having your baby. If you live in

the UK, then the National Health Service (NHS) is your best friend as most of the maternity care is free at the point of use – Yes, it's on the house! We're talking:

- **Antenatal care.** This covers regular check-ups, ultrasounds, blood tests, and other necessary tests. Think of it as a VIP pass to peace of mind. Your partner and you get to see the progress, hear the heartbeat, and ask all those burning questions.

- **Intrapartum care.** Includes labour and delivery services and that sweet hospital stay. This is all about the hands-on support and medical care you and your partner will receive during the actual birth. Think of it as having an all-star medical team ready to guide you through the big moment. They monitor the baby's heart rate, manage pain relief, and ensure everything goes as smoothly as possible.

- **Postnatal care.** Those follow-up appointments and health checks to ensure your little one and partner are thriving. This includes check-ups, breastfeeding support, and making sure everyone's adjusting to the new normal. It's like having a safety net as you figure out this whole parenting gig.

- **Optional Extras.** Though almost everything is covered, you might choose to go the extra mile with optional or private services. Maybe you want those fancy 3D baby scans for extra peace of mind or specialist consultations if you have specific concerns, or you might want to have your baby in a private hospital that offers fancy birthing suites and more personalised care. Just remember, these extras come with a price tag. So, consider this before you start spending those pennies you saved on the NHS.

Health Insurance in the U.S. of A.
It's a bit more complicated if you live across the pond, as navigating healthcare costs during pregnancy can sometimes

feel like trying to solve a Rubik's cube with blindfolds on. But let's try and make it a little less daunting.

Your first step towards mastering the maze of pregnancy-related medical costs is understanding health insurance - your trusted ally and occasional source of headaches. If you have an insurance plan in place, it'll most likely cover most of your pregnancy-related expenses. However, because the specifics can vary widely from plan to plan, I would strongly advise that you take a very close look at the small print to avoid any surprises. Most plans cover:

- **Prenatal Care.** The all-important prenatal visits, ultrasounds, and other fascinating tests to ensure that both mum and baby are in the best possible health, are included in this.

- **Childbirth Care.** This includes hospital stays, labour and delivery, and some postpartum care, but there might still be some out-of-pocket costs. From midwives to doctors and even doulas, as long as you're covered, these folks are there to make sure everything goes smoothly. They'll keep a close eye on both mum and baby, manage pain relief, and guide you through every contraction.

- **Postpartum Care.** This would usually cover follow-up appointments, breastfeeding support, helping mum recover physically and emotionally, and any additional support, but make sure to double-check the small print.

Resources and Lifelines: Freebies and Not-So Freebies
Maybe you're one of those dads who feels uncomfortable when offered a freebie. Well, all I'll say is that if you live in the UK, perhaps now is not the time to be shy or proud, especially when it comes to tapping into NHS lifesavers. They offer resources such as:

- **Midwife-Led Care.** Midwives are like your pregnancy Yoda, offering personalised care, wisdom and support throughout pregnancy and childbirth. They answer all your burning questions and help you feel empowered every step of the way.

- **Local Support Groups.** These are gold mines for advice and moral support. They provide a safe space to share experiences, ask questions, and just vent when needed. It's an opportunity to connect with others who are in the same boat, learning from their journeys and finding a sense of community.

- **The trustworthy NHS Choices.** This is your go-to online resource for all things maternity care, including your rights, services and support to help you through the pregnancy journey. Whether you need tips on healthy eating, advice on managing stress, or just want to know what to expect next, the NHS has got your back (and front and sides).

There are also various forms of financial assistance and benefits available to help with healthcare costs, which I'd advise you not to overlook. They include:

- **Maternity Allowance (MA).** For those who don't qualify for Statutory Maternity Pay (SMP). Whether you're self-employed or your job situation doesn't meet the usual criteria, MA ensures you get the support you deserve. Depending on your circumstances, you could get it for up to 39 weeks, which is some relief when you're juggling baby expenses.

- **Sure Start Maternity Grant.** A one-off payment to help with baby essentials for those who need it most. Whether it's for baby clothes or just stocking up on diapers, this grant can be a real lifesaver.

- **Child Benefit.** Monthly payments to help with the cost of raising your little one. These payments are available to most families, regardless of income. If your child is under 16 (or under 20 if they stay in education), you can make a claim, giving you some long-term financial support as they grow up.

It's a similar scenario in the States. Your insurance plan may have hidden gems waiting to be discovered. But to utilise and maximise these insurance benefits, you need to:

- **Read the Fine Print.** Know your insurance policy inside and out and understand what's covered and what's not. It may be a bit time-consuming, but it is well worth it.

- **Get Pre-Approval.** Always get the green light from your insurer for any non-routine procedures or specialist visits.

- **Know Your "Out-of-Pocket Maximum".** You must familiarise yourself with this term - it will help you avoid unexpected expenses.

It may also be worth exploring the financial support programs available to help cover maternity costs, such as:

- **Medicaid.** If you qualify, it can provide comprehensive coverage for pregnancy-related expenses. It's like hitting the healthcare jackpot.

- **The Children's Health Insurance Program (CHIP).** This offers free or low-cost health coverage to children who are not eligible for Medicaid.

- **Community Programs.** Look for local programs that offer free services, grants and financial aid to help cover medical expenses. It never hurts to ask around.

Navigating maternity expenses can sometimes feel overwhelming, but remember, you're not alone. There are plenty of resources and financial lifelines out there, from government grants to employer benefits to community help. However, it's up to you to take advantage of the available support.

Budgeting for Baby Essentials

Becoming a dad is one of life's most incredible journeys, but let's face it, it's also one of the priciest. Suddenly, you find yourself in the magical universe of baby products, where everything seems both critical and confusing. It's like stepping into a parallel universe where the vocabulary is entirely foreign, and the price tags can make your eyes water. But budgeting for baby essentials doesn't have to be overwhelming. With a bit of planning and some smart shopping, you can get everything you need without breaking the bank. So, grab a hot chocolate, and let's break down how to prepare for your little one's arrival in the most wallet-friendly way possible.

Navigating the Baby Aisle Adventure

When you're knee-deep in the baby aisle, it helps to have a guide to help you make informed decisions on everything from strollers to pacifiers, and no, that guide isn't me. This is where in-depth product reviews and recommendations come in handy. Websites like Consumer Reports offer unbiased baby gear reviews, helping you weigh the pros and cons. Online parenting forums and communities are another goldmine. Sometimes, the best advice comes from those who've been there and done that. Real parents share real experiences, and their insights can be invaluable. It's like having a team of experts in your corner, ready to steer you in the right direction.

What You Really Need

So, what are the must-haves? While it's easy to get swept up in the adorable but not-so-necessary items, focusing on the essentials will save you money and space.

- **Diapers and Wipes.** These are the MVPs of baby essentials. Trust me, you'll go through these faster than you can say "diaper duty." So, stock up, especially during sales, on various sizes because babies grow at lightning speed. And if you're up for some extra laundry, you could consider reusable nappies. As for wipes, they're not just for changing nappies - they'll become your go-to for spills, sticky fingers, and even quick clean-ups on the go. Look for bulk deals to save some cash, and consider eco-friendly options if you're feeling green.

- **A Diaper Bag.** You could call this the ultimate lifesaver. This trusty sidekick is essential for all those on-the-go moments with your little one. Pack it with diapers, wipes, a change of clothes, bottles, and snacks, and don't forget a toy or two for distraction duty. Look for a bag with plenty of compartments to keep things organised and a comfortable strap because you'll be carrying it everywhere.

- **Clothing.** Babies grow faster than you can blink, so don't go overboard. Stick to the basics - onesies, sleepers, and a few cute outfits for special occasions. Comfort is key, so look for soft, stretchy fabrics that are easy to put on and take off. No matter how cute they look, try to avoid clothes with complicated fastenings or too many buttons.

- **Feeding Supplies.** These are the unsung heroes of parenthood. Whether breastfeeding, formula-feeding, or a mix of both, you'll need a few basics. Stock up on bottles, nipples, and a trusty bottle brush for hassle-free cleaning. If breastfeeding is on the agenda, a decent breast pump and some storage bags are must-haves. And don't underestimate the power of a comfy nursing pillow - it'll save your back during those late-night feeds.

- **Cot (Crib) and Bedding.** A safe, comfy cot or crib is a must-have for sweet dreams and safe snoozing. Look for one that meets safety standards and ideally converts into a toddler bed to get more mileage out of your investment. As for bedding, keep it simple and safe - fitted sheets, a couple of sleep sacks or baby blankets, and you're good to go. Avoid overloading with pillows and fluffy stuff to keep your baby's sleep environment secure.

- **Car Seat.** This is non-negotiable. A must-have for every new parent who drives. Safety first, right? You'll need one that's easy to install and adjust and meets the latest safety standards. Trust me, you'll appreciate the convenience during those quick grocery runs or family outings. Plus, with so many options out there, you can find one that fits your car and your budget.

- **Stroller.** A dad's best friend! Look for one that's sturdy, easy to fold, and fits your lifestyle - whether you're into city strolls or off-road adventures. Features like ample storage, a comfy seat, and smooth manoeuvrability will make those outings a breeze. And don't forget, it's got to fit in your car boot!

Stretching Those Coins

Now that we've tied down the basics, let's talk money-saving tips. Here are some tried-and-tested ways to stretch your cash:

- **Sales and Discounts.** Be on the lookout for special offers. They can save you a bundle on baby essentials. Sign up for store newsletters to get the latest deals sent straight to your inbox, and don't hesitate to use coupons. Joining parenting forums can also give you the inside scoop on deals. Seasonal sales and clearance racks are goldmines for finding great bargains on everything from clothes to toys. With some smart shopping and a bit of patience, you can keep your budget intact while still getting everything your baby needs.

- **Online Shopping.** This is a lifesaver for busy parents, and in my opinion, it offers an array of benefits that are often hard to beat. Okay, I may sound slightly biased, but in most cases, shopping online for baby essentials is a more practical and efficient choice for first-time dads. It combines the ease of home shopping, the benefit of consumer reviews and ratings to help make smarter buying decisions, the advantage of a wider selection and better prices, thanks to numerous sales and discounts. And all from the comfort of your home.

- **A Baby Registry.** This is like creating a wish list of all the baby essentials you need, and it helps your friends and family know exactly what to get you. Not only does it save you money, but it also ensures you get items you'll actually use. Be sure to include a mix of must-haves and nice-to-haves, and don't forget to add some affordable options for every budget. Plus, many stores offer perks just for signing up.

- **Bulk Buying.** Alright, dads, let's talk about the power of bulk buying. Buying in bulk is the way to go when it comes to essentials like nappies, wipes, and formula. Not only do you get more bang for your buck, but you also save yourself from those last-minute store runs. Sign up for warehouse memberships or online deals to get big packs at discounted prices. Just make sure you've got the storage space at home to keep everything neatly organised.

DIY Essentials. Time to unleash your inner handyman! Getting crafty can save you some serious cash while adding a personal touch to your baby's gear. There are endless ways to get creative, from making your own baby food to

DIY nursery décor. Not only will you save money, but you'll also have some fun and make unique items for your little one. Plus, you get the added bonus of feeling like a super-dad who can tackle anything.

- **Second-Hand Savings.** This isn't for everyone, but if it's for you, this could be a treasure trove. Babies outgrow stuff so quickly, which means you can get some amazing deals on fairly used items. Whether clothes, toys, furniture or other gear, second-hand shops and online marketplaces are your best friends. Not only does it save you a ton of money, but it's also eco-friendly - talk about a win-win! Don't shy away from hand-me-downs from friends and family that are in excellent condition. It's all about getting great quality for less and being budget-conscious.

Make Smart Choices

Not every item needs to be top-of-the-line, but some are worth spending a bit more on. By knowing where to splurge and finding clever ways to save, you can keep your budget in check. Here's a quick guide:

- **Smart Splurges.** While saving is great, some items are worth the extra investment. Think about splurging on a high-quality car seat and cot (crib) - safety and comfort are uncompromisable for your little one. A good stroller that's easy to manoeuvre and folds up in a flash can save you a lot of hassle. And you could add a reliable baby monitor to your splurge basket for that extra peace of mind. These splurges can make life easier and ensure your baby's safety and comfort.

- **Smart Saves.** When it comes to baby gear, not everything needs to be top-of-the-line. Save on items like baby clothes, toys, and even some nursery décor - babies outgrow these things so quickly! If it's an acceptable option, consider shopping second-hand or accepting hand-me-downs from friends and family. You'll be amazed at the excellent quality you can find without spending a fortune.

Budgeting for baby essentials is all about balance. With some research, planning and a bit of savvy shopping, you can handle this like a pro. So, take a deep breath, and remember that it's not all about designer clothes and the latest gadgets. It's more to do with choosing what's safe, practical, and within your budget. Whatever the case, your baby will bring you joy that's worth every single penny.

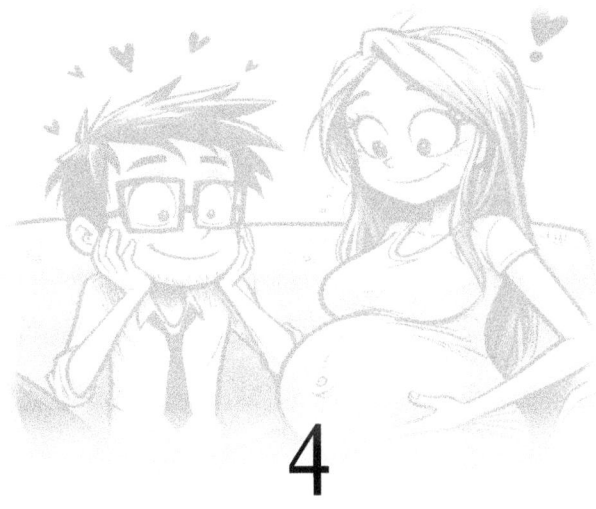

4

The Nine-Month Adventure
Navigating the Pregnancy Journey

From the initial excitement of finding out you're going to be a dad to feeling those first baby kicks to the final weeks before your baby arrives, each pregnancy stage brings its own unique experiences and challenges. Knowing what to expect in each trimester can help you support your partner through the highs and lows and actively participate in this exciting journey.

Journeying Through Trimesters

Pregnancy is a wild ride, a nine-month adventure where each trimester brings its own set of surprises and milestones. Let's take a brief look at the common changes that happen during each trimester.

First Trimester: Adjusting to New Realities
The first trimester is a time of breathtaking changes as your partner's body gears up for the momentous task of growing a

tiny human. This stage is often marked by fatigue and nausea, those delightful symptoms that make getting out of bed feel like running a marathon. Your partner's body is working overtime, and her energy levels might be at an all-time low. It's all about adjusting to the new realities of pregnancy, finding a rhythm amidst the chaos, and supporting her as she navigates these challenging early days. As your partner adapts, so do you, learning to anticipate her needs and offer a helping hand when needed.

Second Trimester: The Sweet Spot

Then comes the second trimester, often referred to as the "sweet spot" of pregnancy. Energy levels start to pick up, and your partner might find herself feeling more like her old self. It's a time when many women experience a renewed sense of vitality, and those first flutters of baby movement can bring a sense of wonder and connection. It's also when physical changes become more pronounced, with the baby bump making its grand debut. This is your cue to get proactive. Attending antenatal (prenatal) classes together can provide valuable insights and prepare you both for what's to come. These classes are not just about breathing techniques; they're about equipping you both with the knowledge to handle the unexpected with grace and humour.

Third Trimester: The Countdown

The third trimester is the final countdown. As the excitement of the approaching due date builds, so do the preparations. This is the time to get those nesting instincts into high gear. Preparing the nursery becomes a top priority, turning that spare room into a cosy haven for your little one. And don't forget to pack your hospital bag. Having everything ready to go can save you from last-minute scrambles and ensure that you're prepared for the big day. Think of it as packing for the most important trip of your life - a journey into parenthood.

Tracking the Bump

Tracking your baby's development is more than just a

weekly ritual; it's a way to stay connected with the little life growing inside your partner. Weekly development apps can be a fun way to see how your baby is changing from the size of a peach to a watermelon. These updates can be a source of excitement and anticipation, bringing you closer to the reality of becoming a parent. Reading monthly pregnancy guides can also help you understand the changes your partner is experiencing, keeping you informed and ready to offer support. It's about staying engaged and involved, even when things get hectic.

Navigating the Twists and Turns Together

Feeling a bit anxious about the changes your partner might face is normal, but being informed can make a huge difference. From morning sickness and fatigue to back pain and mood swings, being clued up on these concerns means you can be the supportive partner she needs. So, let's break down what to expect and how to navigate these bumps in the road together. Your partner will appreciate your extra effort, and you'll feel more confident as you tackle the ups and downs side by side.

- **Morning Sickness.** From the day I met my wife over 33 years ago, she and fried plantain - which we call "dodo" in my local dialect - had been inseparable. I'm not exaggerating when I say she'd find it hard to survive without it. So, imagine my surprise when she said she didn't want to eat, smell, or even see dodo as the mere whiff now sent her sprinting to the bathroom. Well, welcome to the world of the infamous, not-so-glamorous morning sickness. Despite its name, it can strike anytime, day or night. Your partner might feel queasy, tired, and just plain miserable, and that's where you come in. Keep the house stocked with ginger tea, crackers, and other tummy-friendly snacks. Encourage her to eat small, frequent meals and stay hydrated. Offer a listening ear, and try to keep things light-hearted to help her through the rough patches. Your patience, sympathy, support and understanding can make all the difference.

- **Pre-eclampsia.** If not managed properly, this condition can be dangerous for both mum and baby. It is characterised by high blood pressure. Watch out for these symptoms: severe headaches, vision changes, hand and face swelling, and sudden weight gain. You must contact your doctor immediately if your partner experiences any of these. Your role is to stay calm, be supportive, and help her keep track of any symptoms. Regular prenatal check-ups are essential for monitoring her blood pressure and catching any signs early. Encouraging her to rest, reduce stress, and follow the doctor's advice can go a long way in managing this condition.

- **Gestational Diabetes.** This can develop when your partner's body has trouble managing blood sugar levels. It sounds daunting, but it can be managed effectively by taking the right steps. It's important to follow the doctor's advice, which might include dietary changes, regular blood sugar monitoring, and regular physical activity, such as walking. Encourage her to eat healthy, balanced meals that are low in sugar and high in nutrients. Join her in these healthy eating habits; it's easier when you're in it together. Managing gestational diabetes is a team effort, and your support and understanding can make a big difference in keeping both mum and baby healthy.

- **Premature (Preterm) Labour.** This occurs when your partner goes into labour before 37 weeks of pregnancy. The signs include regular contractions, lower back pain, and changes in vaginal discharge. If you notice any of these signs, contact your doctor immediately. It's always better to be safe than sorry. Staying calm and collected is key -

you're her rock in this moment. Encourage her to rest and stay hydrated while you make the necessary calls. Having a go-bag packed and ready can also ease some of the stress if you need to make a quick trip to the hospital. Remember, catching preterm labour early can make a significant difference.

- **Pregnancy Brain.** Pregnancy brain isn't a figment of imagination or an old wives' tale; it's a real phenomenon that many expectant mothers face. According to the experts, increased levels of progesterone and estrogen during the whirlwind of critical developments in the first trimester are believed to contribute to this temporary forgetfulness. Couple that with your partner's body using up a ton of energy to grow that little one; it's no surprise that she might sometimes forget why she walked into a room. To help out, you can create shared to-do lists so you're both on the same page and set reminders for vital appointments. It's a small gesture, but it shows you've got her back. Listen to her without being judgmental, and gently remind her of things without sounding annoyed. A little kindness and a high dose of empathy can really go a long way. Also, make sure you keep the communication lines open - talking about your feelings and challenges can help both of you feel more connected and manage the ups and downs together during this phase.

- **Fatigue.** Pregnancy can be draining for your partner. She's growing a tiny human, after all! That means her body is working overtime, so fatigue is totally normal. She might feel like she's running on empty most days, especially as the baby grows and demands more energy. So, being the loving husband that you are, helping out with household chores, cooking meals, or just letting her nap whenever she needs to are things she will appreciate. Encourage her to take breaks and pamper herself a little. Also, simple things like prepping a cosy spot with pillows and blankets, making her favourite snacks, or just being there to lend a hand can have a huge impact.

- **Back Pain.** As your partner's belly grows, the additional weight and shifting centre of gravity put extra strain on her back. This can lead to severe discomfort, and she'll need your support. Start with simple solutions like encouraging good posture - remind her to stand up straight and use a supportive chair if she's sitting for long periods. A pregnancy pillow can work wonders at night, providing that much-needed support while she sleeps. Gentle back massages are a great way to help ease the tension, and bonus points if you use some soothing lotion or oil. You might also consider joining her in some light stretching exercises; apart from helping to strengthen those back muscles and provide relief, this is a great way to bond and stay active together. If the pain gets too intense, don't hesitate to ask your midwife for advice. Being proactive and supportive shows your partner that you're there every step of the way.

- **Heartburn.** As your partner's belly grows and her digestive system gets squished, heartburn can become a regular, unwelcome visitor. It feels like swallowing fire, and it's a common complaint in pregnancy. Encourage her to eat smaller, more frequent meals rather than big ones and avoid spicy, fatty, or acidic foods. Asking her to stay upright after meals can also help - no lying down right after eating. And propping up her head with an extra pillow while she sleeps can also do wonders. Having some pregnancy-safe antacids on hand can provide quick relief, but always check with your doctor first. Dealing with heartburn is tough, but she'll get through it with your support.

- **Swollen Feet and Ankles.** As your partner's body adjusts to accommodate the growing baby, it's not uncommon for her to experience some swelling, especially in her feet and ankles. This can be uncomfortable and sometimes even painful. Encourage her to put her feet up whenever possible to reduce swelling. A little footrest or a stack of pillows can help. Ensure she's staying well-hydrated - drinking plenty of water helps flush out excess fluids. Gentle, soothing foot massages can also provide some much-needed relief. If she's on her feet a lot, remind her to take breaks and sit down for a bit. Comfortable, supportive shoes are a must, so maybe treat her to a new pair that will keep her feet happy. And if the swelling gets worse, don't hesitate to call your doctor.

- **Mood Swings.** With her hormones in overdrive during pregnancy, your partner might experience everything from joy and excitement to tears and frustration, sometimes all within a few hours. It's completely normal, but it can be tricky to navigate. You need to be the steady anchor. Be patient and understanding, even when the mood swings catch you off guard. Listen intently and offer a reassuring hug or some comforting words. Encourage her to talk about her feelings, and don't take the emotional ups and downs personally. If she's feeling particularly stressed, suggest relaxation techniques like deep breathing or a calming walk together. A little bit of humour can also help lighten the mood - just be sensitive to her feelings and know when it's the right time for a laugh.

- **Cravings and Aversions.** Your partner's taste buds might go wild, making her yearn for the strangest food combos or completely rejecting her once-favourite dishes. This can be both amusing and challenging. One day, it's dodo and stew; the next day, the mere smell of tea sends her running. This is all thanks to those pregnancy hormones working their magic. Embrace the quirks with a sense of humour and an open mind. If she's craving something unusual (and safe), do your best to satisfy that craving – a midnight run to the fridge for pineapple chops, anyone? On the flip side, respect her aversions; if she suddenly can't stand the sight of chicken, find alternative meals that won't make her queasy. Keep a stash of her favourite snacks handy and be ready to whip up some spontaneous culinary concoctions. Once again, showing your support through these foodie ups and downs helps strengthen your bond.

- **Frequent Urination.** As the baby grows and your partner's uterus expands, it puts extra pressure on her bladder, making her feel like she needs to go all the time. This can be super annoying, especially at night when it interrupts her sleep. Your mission? Be understanding and supportive. Remind her to stay hydrated, but suggest she drinks more during the day and less in the evening to minimise nighttime trips. Help her create a comfortable bathroom setup - maybe even a nightlight to make those midnight runs easier. Encourage her to wear loose, comfortable clothing that doesn't put extra pressure on her bladder.

- **Leg Cramps.** These sudden, painful muscle spasms, often occurring at night, can really disrupt your partner's sleep and comfort. Encourage her to stretch her legs regularly throughout the day, especially before bedtime - simple calf stretches can work wonders. Make sure she stays hydrated, as dehydration can sometimes trigger cramps. A warm soak before bed can help relax her muscles and make it easier to fall asleep. During a cramp, gently massage the affected area to help ease the pain and encourage her to flex her foot - pulling her toes towards her shin can often bring relief. A balanced diet rich in calcium and magnesium is a good option, as deficiencies in these minerals can contribute to cramps. Whether fetching a glass of water or being there with a comforting hand, your support makes these uncomfortable moments more bearable.

Through the joys and scares of pregnancy, being supportive, informed, and proactive can make a world of difference for both mum and baby. You're an integral part of this pregnancy journey, so see it as a time of growth, change, and preparation. Remember that each pregnancy phase is a step closer to meeting your little one. Keep learning, asking questions, and, most importantly, be there every step of the way.

Nine months of waiting, oh, what a ride,
From the first trimester to little baby's cry.
Cravings and mood swings, all day and night,
You're there for each moment, holding her tight.

Ultrasounds and baby kicks, what a joy to see,
Planning the nursery, dreaming of who they'll be.
Late-night snacks and midnight talks,
Together, you stroll on those pregnancy walks.

From tiny flutters to a growing bump,
Feeling that tiny heart pump.
You've got the laughs and a heart full of cheer,
So, get ready, Dad, your baby's almost here!

~ akin.o ~

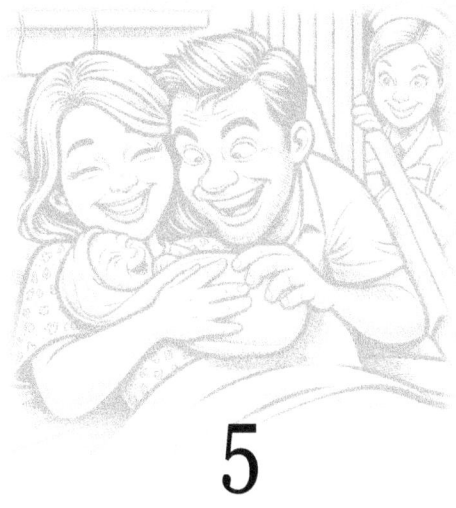

5

The Big Push
From Bump to Baby

Imagine yourself in the heart of a busy hospital corridor, tightly clutching a crumpled piece of paper, with your birth plan scribbled all over it, as if your life depended on it. The air around you buzzes with expectation and the faint aroma of antiseptic. Welcome to the labour ward, the place where chaos and miracles coexist.

The Birth Plan: Your Delivery Blueprint

As you prepare to welcome your tiny human into the world, having a birth plan can be an ace in the hole. It's like having a roadmap for the journey ahead, even if you end up taking a few detours along the way. A birth plan is more than just a list of preferences; it's a communication tool that helps ensure everyone's on the same page when the big moment arrives. Think of it as your dialogue starter with the medical team, a way to express your and your partner's desires and concerns clearly.

Crafting Your Dream Delivery

Crafting a comprehensive birth plan involves more than jotting down a few bullet points. It's about considering the elements that matter most to you and your partner. Perhaps you've got a specific request for pain management or a particular birthing position in mind. Discussing these options with your midwife beforehand is crucial. It ensures that your desires are feasible and align with medical best practices. This conversation also helps set realistic expectations, allowing you to navigate the delivery day with confidence and clarity.

Syncing Up with the Birth Team

As a first-time dad, the labour ward (delivery room) might seem like uncharted territory, but where possible, building a rapport with the medical team can make the experience less daunting. Start by introducing yourself and, as mentioned earlier, sharing your birth plan preferences; a friendly "hello" and a warm smile can go a long way. Understand the roles of the key players - from the obstetrician to the midwives and nurses. This way, you'll feel more at ease and know who to turn to when things get intense. Building this connection ensures everyone is on the same page, making the experience smoother and more favourable for your partner.

Expecting the Unexpected

Of course, birth plans are not set in stone. Babies have a knack for being unpredictable, and sometimes, plans need to change. That's why contingency planning is essential. Prepare for potential changes by understanding that flexibility and adaptability are your best friends. Mentally rehearse scenarios where quick decisions might be needed, like opting for a C-section if complications arise. It's about being prepared to pivot, ensuring that both your partner and baby receive the best care possible. Remember, the ultimate goal is a healthy mum and baby, which sometimes means adjusting your original plan.

Embracing Your Birth Duties

So, it's finally here. The grand finale of pregnancy, where all the anticipation and preparation come to a head. You're about to witness the miracle of birth, and you've got a front-row seat like no other. The only difference is that you won't be sitting down because you have a vital role to play.

The Perfect Birthing Buddy
As a dad-to-be, your presence in the delivery room is more than symbolic. It's a chance to be your partner's rock, the calming voice amidst the whirlwind. Providing emotional and physical support can make a world of difference, and that's where you come in. Words of encouragement can be incredibly powerful. A simple "You've got this" or "You're doing great" can give your partner the reassurance she needs. Helping your partner with breathing exercises to manage the pain and keeping her calm and focused, your role is to comfort her and make sure she has everything she needs. Remember, you're her perfect support.

A Gentle Touch
Don't underestimate the power of a simple touch. A gentle massage, a light touch on the back or shoulders, or even applying pressure or a warm cloth on your partner's lower back can be quite soothing and help ease tension. Encouraging hydration and energy intake is vital, too. Offer sips of water or an electrolyte drink, and keep some light snacks on hand. They're sure to come in handy. Your role is simply to help her stay calm, comfortable and distracted; you'd be surprised at how a walk around the block or an episode of her favourite series could work wonders.

The "C" Word
What would we do without it? Just like in most areas, communication is your magic wand during labour. Clear and effective communication between you, your partner and

the medical staff ensures everyone is on the same page. Don't hesitate to ask questions if something isn't clear. If there's medical jargon flying around, asking for clarification can help you both understand what's happening. Advocating for your partner's needs and preferences is crucial. If she's unable to communicate her wishes, step up and ensure her voice is heard. It's all about being her voice when she needs it most. Remember, your role is to be her champion, cheerleader, and advocate, all rolled into one.

The Labour Ward: Tips and Need-to-Knows

The labour ward is a place of incredible emotion and energy, where every moment counts. Being prepared, supportive, and attentive can make a world of difference as you welcome your little one into the world.

Essential Hospital Bag Tips

As the big day approaches, you might find yourself wondering what exactly to pack for the hospital. Start with the basics:

- Pack some snacks to keep your energy up during those potentially long hours

- A phone with a charger is a must-have for those crucial updates to family and friends

- Don't forget a change of clothes, toiletries, and nursing bras for your partner

- Essential documents should also be within reach – including maternity notes, insurance cards and any necessary paperwork depending on where you're having your baby

- For added comfort, you may bring your own pillow or

blanket, a music playlist to set the mood, and a camera to capture those first precious moments

The truth is that what you put in the bag depends solely on you and your partner. Personalising your hospital bag to meet your and your partner's needs ensures you're not caught off guard when the time finally comes.

Labour Ward Etiquette
Understanding the etiquette of the delivery room is key to maintaining a supportive environment. Respecting the medical staff is paramount. They're there to ensure both mum and baby are safe, so following their instructions is essential. It's easy to get caught up in the moment, but avoid unnecessary distractions like excessive phone use. This is a time to be present, engaged, and focused on your partner's needs. Your attention is a gift, one that shows her she's your priority.

Stay Calm Under Pressure
Staying calm under pressure is easier said than done, but it's vital. Labour can be intense, and your partner might look to you for reassurance. So, it is important that you know your personal stress signals, whether it's a racing heart or a clenched jaw, and take steps to manage them. Find what works for you: a quick walk in the hallway, a few moments of quiet reflection, stress-reduction techniques like deep breathing, or visualising a peaceful place; know what works for you. Being a calm presence and maintaining your composure in the room provides invaluable support for your partner. Even a simple smile can convey the strength and support she needs.

Labour Unveiled

Labour typically unfolds in three main stages, each with its unique rhythm and tempo, each with its own set of challenges and milestones.

The First Stage: From Warm-Up to Whirlwind

This is when things start to get real. There's an air of excitement, anticipation and unpredictability. It all kicks off with early labour.

- **Early labour.** This is the warm-up act. It is the longest phase and can last from a few hours to several days when the cervix dilates from 0 to 6 centimetres. Your partner might experience mild and irregular contractions akin to period cramps, which gradually become stronger and more regular. She might feel a bit restless or notice some backache. It's like the body sending out little reminders that showtime is near. As labour progresses, it transitions into active labour.

- **Active Labour.** This is when things start getting real. Contractions become more frequent and intense as the cervix dilates from 6 to 10 centimetres. It's time to head to the hospital. You'll know it's active labour when the contractions occur every few minutes and last between 45 to 60 seconds.

The Second Stage: The Final Push

This is where things really heat up as your partner's body prepares to bring your little one into the world. It's intense, it's exhilarating, and, I'd say, a true test of strength and determination.

- **Transition.** This phase is the crescendo. The cervix dilates to 10 centimetres, and contractions are at their peak intensity and frequency. Though it is often the shortest, it is the most intense part of labour. It's a whirlwind, but remember, you're preparing to meet your little one.

- **Pushing.** This stage kicks in when the cervix is fully dilated and ultimately ends with the birth of your little one. Pushing can last from a few minutes to several hours. Please do your best to encourage your partner to find a comfortable position and to listen to her body and the medical team's guidance. Since you can't push, your job is to be actively present, offering support and motivation.

- **Delivery.** Once your baby's head crowns, the rest of the body follows quickly. This is the moment you've been waiting for! It's an emotional and exhilarating experience. Be prepared for a surge of emotions and a lot of activity in the delivery room.

The Third Stage: The After-Party

The hard part is over; now it's time for the final chapter: the afterbirth.

- **Afterbirth.** After your little one is born, mild contractions continue to help deliver the placenta. This usually happens within 30 minutes after birth. It is usually brief and ensures the entire placenta is expelled to prevent complications.

Don't forget that communicating with the healthcare team and effective pain management techniques also play significant roles during labour.

Baby's First Hello

The moment you've been waiting for is finally here. After what felt like a marathon, you get to meet this tiny human who's been camping out in your partner's belly. It's a magical and surreal experience to see and hold your little one for the first time. As you cradle that tiny bundle of joy, take a deep breath and soak it all in. The first cry, those little fingers grasping yours – it's pure magic. Whether you're snapping photos or just savouring the moment, know that this is the beginning of something really special.

First Steps into Dadhood

As you step into the realm of initial baby care, there's a sense of responsibility and connection that comes with each task. If you're up for it, cutting the umbilical cord can be a profound experience – it's like officially welcoming your baby into the world. And then there's the first diaper change, a rite of passage for every new dad. Approach it with humour and patience because, let's face it, you're both learning. These first care tasks are more than chores; they're moments of bonding where you start to understand the unique rhythm of caring for your child.

Getting Acquainted

Your first interactions with your baby are the foundation of your relationship. Talking softly to them as you hold them in your arms helps them recognise your voice and presence. These early moments of holding and comforting are where you begin to forge a bond that will last a lifetime. It's about creating a sense of security and warmth, letting your baby know they're loved and cherished. This connection is a two-way street because you'll find that the simple act of holding your baby close calms your own nerves, too, reinforcing that you're in this together.

Capture Every Moment

As you hold your newborn for the first time, capturing these early moments becomes a treasure trove of memories. Snapping a quick photo or recording a short video of your baby's first cry isn't just about preserving a moment - it's about encapsulating the raw, beautiful chaos of birth. It's these little snippets of time that you'll look back on, standing on the sidelines of those first steps or their high school graduation. Consider jotting down your initial thoughts or feelings in a journal, something to revisit on those sleepless nights when you wonder how it all began. Documenting the time of birth and those tiny details like weight and length may seem trivial now, but trust me, future you will thank you for it.

Baby's First Check-Up

Be prepared for the standard post-delivery medical checks and procedures. The APGAR score, a quick assessment of your baby's health, might sound intimidating, but it's just a routine check. Baby screening tests will follow, aimed at ensuring your little one is off to a healthy start. Understanding these procedures can ease any anxiety you might have, allowing you to focus on what truly matters - being there for your partner and baby.

Remember that the first moments with your baby are just the beginning - an introduction to a lifetime of love, laughter, and learning. Cherish every moment.

It's big push day, oh what a scene,
You're by her side, feeling so keen.
With a deep breath and a loving smile,
You're cheering her on, "You've got this, girl!"

From "You can do it!" to "Just one more!"
You're there for her, a hundred percent and more.
Holding her hand, wiping her brow,
A team together, you've made it somehow.

With a final push and a joyous cry,
Your little one's here; how time flies.
Teary-eyed, full of pride,
Are you ready for this wild, beautiful ride?

~ akin.o ~

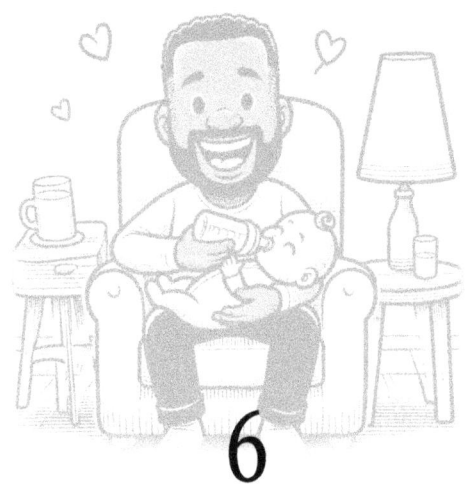

6

Baby Bootcamp ~ Phase I
Surviving Newborn Chaos, Feeds, and Naps

So, your little bundle of joy has finally arrived, and as you hold them, it's hard to believe that just a few days ago, they were snugly nestled in your partner's belly. Welcome to the newborn phase - a time of incredible joy, sleepless nights, and moments that will test your ingenuity and patience. Think of this phase as a crash course in baby wrangling. It's about embracing the mess, the magic, and the mayhem that comes with being a new dad. The experts say that the official length of this phase is about 28 days, but personally, I think it lasts a bit longer. So, take the following two chapters as your backstage pass to what you need to know about surviving and thriving during the first few months.

Embrace the Unpredictability

Bringing your baby home is a milestone like no other. It's the moment when theory meets reality, and you realise that those parenting books only scratched the surface. Adjusting to life with a baby requires a shift in priorities and routines. Everything revolves around this tiny human who demands your attention at all hours. It's a bit like starting a new job without any training, but the stakes are infinitely higher. Your world suddenly revolves around feedings, diaper changes, and soothing cries. It's a beautiful chaos, one that takes time to navigate. The key is embracing the unpredictability, knowing it's okay to feel a little overwhelmed as you find your footing.

Don't Sweat the Small Stuff
I still have a pretty vivid memory of being in the trenches of the newborn phase. I quickly realised that trying to maintain my pre-baby routine was a recipe for disaster. Instead, I had to embrace the chaos by re-prioritising my tasks. I learned to let go of the small stuff and focus on what truly mattered - being present for my wife and baby. By adjusting my expectations and accepting the unpredictability, I found a new rhythm that worked for me and the family. The bottom line is that thriving in the early weeks is all about adaptability and teamwork.

Growing into Dadhood
Adjusting to life with a newborn is an ongoing process, filled with trial and error. There will be moments of triumph, like mastering the art of the quick diaper change, and moments of doubt, like wondering if you'll ever feel rested again. But through it all, remember that you're equipped with the most important tool of all - LOVE. It's the driving force that will guide you, even on the most challenging days. As you embrace the ups and downs, know that each day is a step forward, a chance to grow into the role of a lifetime.

The Round-the-Clock Buffet

Feeding your newborn is one of the most intimate and crucial aspects of early parenting, but here's one thing you should know. They may have tiny tummies, but feeding them is like an all-you-can-eat buffet that never closes because they need to eat frequently.

Breast, Bottle or Both

Whether you're breastfeeding, bottle feeding, or doing a combo, there are a few need-to-knows when it comes to navigating the world of round-the-clock feedings with your little gourmet.

Breastfeeding. This is nature's way of providing the essential nutrients and antibodies needed to boost your baby's immune system. We all know you can't breastfeed, but you can play a huge role in making it a successful experience. Start by being the ultimate cheerleader - encourage and reassure your partner during those sleepless nights and tricky latch moments. Help with the prep work by fetching water, snacks, or that favourite pillow for extra comfort. You can also handle diaper changes, burping, and soothing the baby after feedings to give your partner a break. And don't forget, skin-to-skin cuddles with your little one are not just for mums - those moments will help you bond with the baby and give mum a rest. Your support and involvement can make all the difference in the world! Even though breastfeeding is like nature's perfect meal plan, it has its own hurdles. There are the upsides...

- **All About Nutrition.** Breast milk is the perfect blend of protein, vitamins, and fat your baby needs to grow. Plus, it's easier on their tiny tummies as it's much easier to digest than formula.

- **Immune System Boost.** Breast milk antibodies help your little one fight off viruses and bacteria, lowering the risk of infections and staying healthy.

- **Health Perks for Mum.** Breastfeeding can help your

partner lose baby weight faster and is said to lower the risk of certain cancers. It also releases oxytocin, which helps your partner's body recover after childbirth.

- **Cost Savings.** Breastfeeding can save money by reducing the need for formula and related feeding supplies.

- **Ready and Convenient.** Breast milk is always ready. No bottles to prepare, no formula to mix. Your milk is always on tap and at the perfect temperature.

And the downsides:

- **The Ouch Factor.** Your partner may experience sore nipples, engorged breasts, and the occasional blocked duct, which can be pretty uncomfortable.

- **Diet Detective.** Your partner must watch what she eats as some foods can affect your baby. This could mean no more spicy burritos or extra coffee, at least for now.

- **Time and Patience.** Breastfeeding can be time-consuming and demanding, especially in the beginning when your baby needs to be fed often.

- **Public Feeding.** Your partner might not feel comfy breastfeeding in public, and finding a private spot can be tricky.

- **Sharing the Load.** Breastfeeding can make it harder to hand over feeding duties, making it tough to get a break or some alone time.

Bottle Feeding. Getting in on feeding duties can be a fantastic way to bond with your little one and give mum a well-deserved break. First off, make sure you've got the right supplies - bottles, nipples, and formula. Take charge of sterilising the bottles and nipples, and if you're preparing the bottles, ensure they are done according to the instructions - accurate measurements are crucial. Get into a routine that works for you and your baby. Find a comfy spot for feeding time, and don't rush - enjoy these moments of closeness. After feeding, burp your baby gently to help them release any trapped air. And remember, skin-to-skin contact isn't just for mum; holding your baby close can be a magical bonding experience. There are plenty of perks when it comes to bottle feeding, but it's not without its challenges. There's the great stuff...

- **Shared Feeding Duties.** Bottle feeding lets everyone join in on the fun. Whether it's you, grandma, or anyone else, anyone can help feed the baby, giving mum a much-needed and creating bonding moments for everyone.

- **Flexibility.** You can easily keep track of exactly how much your baby is drinking, and it allows for a more flexible and predictable feeding schedule

- **No Diet Drama.** With formula, your partner doesn't have to worry about the issue of what she eats affecting the baby. Formula is designed to provide all necessary nutrients. So, she may not need to avoid that extra spicy curry or that glass of wine.

- **Public Feeding Made Easy.** You might feel more comfortable feeding your baby with a bottle in public without the need to find a private spot for breastfeeding.

- **Consistent Nutrition:** Formula is designed to be nutritionally complete, so you know they're getting a balanced diet - all the necessary vitamins and minerals.

And the not-so-great stuff:

- **Cha-Ching.** Formula can be pricey, and the costs add up. Plus, you'll need to buy bottles, nipples, and all the other feeding and cleaning supplies.

- **Prep Time.** Bottles need to be washed, sterilised, and prepared, which can take up quite a bit of time, especially during those nighttime feedings.

- **Missing Immunity Boost.** Formula doesn't have the natural antibodies that breast milk has, so babies might not get that extra immune protection.

- **Tummy Troubles.** Your baby may have difficulty digesting formula more than breast milk, leading to gas or constipation.

- **Eco Impact.** There's more waste involved with formula feeding due to the manufacturing, packaging, and disposal of formula containers, bottles and other feeding supplies.

Both breastfeeding and formula feeding have their unique benefits and challenges. The most important thing is to choose what works best for your partner, your baby. Everyone's situation is different; there's no one-size-fits-all answer.

Hunger Cues

Recognising when your baby is hungry is like deciphering a secret baby language, and it's key to keeping those tiny tummies happy. From rooting (turning their head towards your hand) and lip-smacking to sucking on their hands and a good old cry, your little one has a variety of ways to say, "Feed me!" By the way, crying can be a late hunger cue, so try to catch the earlier signs. You can ensure smoother feeding times and a more content baby by tuning in to these signals. Remember, mastering hunger cues is also a fantastic way to bond with your little one and build your confidence as a hands-on dad.

Cluster Feeding

This stage, where your baby wants to feed more frequently than usual, can feel like a marathon of nursing or bottle sessions. But don't worry, your little one is simply gearing up for those big developmental leaps, and they need those extra calories to fuel their journey, or maybe it's merely their way of boosting your partner's milk supply. As you navigate these intense feeding sessions, remember that your support and presence mean the world to both mum and baby. Keep the snacks, water, and entertainment within arm's reach, embrace the cuddle time, stay patient, and know that you're playing a vital role in your baby's growth and well-being.

Surviving the Buffet

Feeding your baby is a round-the-clock commitment. It doesn't always go smoothly, and that's okay. You might encounter challenges like colic or reflux, where your baby seems fussy or uncomfortable after eating, or you might face issues with the little one latching on correctly. Though these can be distressing, there are ways to address them. If you and your partner are struggling, don't hesitate to seek guidance and reassurance from a lactation consultant or your paediatricians. They're like the superheroes of baby nutrition, armed with knowledge and experience. Embrace the chaos, take shifts where possible, and remind yourself that this phase won't last forever. Every feed is a step towards your baby's healthy growth and a chance to bond. You've got this!

Sleep,... or the Lack Thereof

Sleep is a hot commodity during the newborn phase. In fact, it is said to be the elusive dream for every new parent. You'll find yourself perfecting the art of napping while standing or discovering a newfound appreciation for a good cup of coffee. Nights blur into days, and the concept of uninterrupted sleep becomes a distant memory. But don't worry; it won't last forever. It's only a phase! So, in the meantime, you need to figure out your baby's sleep patterns, create a sleep-friendly environment and maybe catch a few winks while you're at it.

Your Baby's Sleep Patterns

One of the first things you'll notice about your baby is their unique sleep patterns. It won't take long before you realise they run on their own schedule. They snooze a lot, typically for 16 – 17 hours, but not in long stretches and, most times, not when you want them to. Your little one will cycle through active and quiet sleep phases:

- Active sleep might involve twitching, rapid eye movement, or little noises.

- Quiet sleep is when they're more still and peaceful.

Knowing these signs can help you adjust your expectations and cope with broken sleep. Adapting your routine to their needs is key, so keep an eye on those sleepy cues.

Safe Sleep Practices

Safety first! Creating a sleep-friendly environment for your little one's safety and comfort is crucial. Start with a firm mattress in a safety-approved cot, keeping the sleep space minimalistic - free from pillows, blankets and toys - and always put your baby to sleep on their back to reduce the Sudden Infant Death Syndrome (SIDS) risk. A sleep sack or swaddle can reduce the startle reflex and also help your baby feel secure. You might think your baby needs complete silence, but a little white noise, the hum of a fan or a gentle lullaby can work wonders, mimicking the sounds of the womb and helping them settle. It also creates a soothing backdrop, encouraging longer stretches of sleep.

Surviving Sleep Deprivation

Sleep deprivation is the unwelcome guest that accompanies

every newborn baby, turning even the most mundane tasks into Herculean feats. It's tough, but you can handle it. Stay hydrated, eat well, and cut yourself some slack - household chores can wait. Prioritise rest so you can be the best version of yourself for your partner and baby. Sleep is not a luxury - it's a necessity for survival. It is important to sneak in naps whenever possible to survive the newborn phase, and here are a few tips to help:

- **Nap When the Baby Naps.** It's classic advice for a reason. Like I said earlier, forget about chores and rest when your baby does, even if it's just for a few precious minutes.

- **Establish a Consistent Sleep Routine.** This can signal to your baby that it's wind-down time. The predictability of a calming bedtime routine, which could include a gentle massage, a warm bath, or a quiet story, can help them associate certain activities with sleep. Helping your baby know the difference between day and night is also important. During the day, keep the lights bright and engage in active play. At night, dim the lights to cue their internal clock for rest. This will help regulate their sleep cycle and would definitely do your sleep routine a favour.

- **Share Nighttime Duties.** Embrace the power of teamwork. You and your partner should take turns with nighttime feedings and diaper changes. This way, both of you can get longer stretches of sleep.

- **Create a Calming Environment.** Make your bedroom a sleep haven. Use blackout curtains and white noise machines, and keep the room cool.

- **Accept Help:** If trustworthy friends or family offer to watch baby, then maybe you should take them up on their offer and try to catch that extra nap.

Remind yourself that this phase is temporary. Your baby

will eventually develop a more predictable sleep pattern, but until then, hang in there, take turns, and cherish those quiet moments when your little one is peacefully sleeping. You will come out on the other side, even on four hours of sleep!

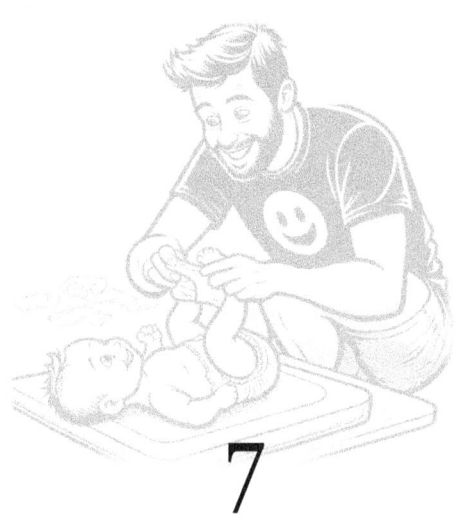

7

Baby Bootcamp ~ Phase II
Diapering, Bathing and Soothing Secrets

You've already learnt the ropes of feeding and sleeping. So, why not take a few extra steps and become a pro in diapering, bathing and soothing, too – all while running on very little sleep? I know it's intense, but you'll soon find yourself becoming a pro at things you never imagined, and those sweet moments with your baby will make it all worthwhile. So, once again, enjoy the mess, the magic, and the mayhem that comes with being a new dad.

Diapering 101: Handling the Mess with Ease

With your baby in one hand and a diaper in the other, it's time to confidently tackle the world of diapers. Diaper duty could be referred to as the unsung hero of parenthood. Though it can be a bit messy, it doesn't mean it can't be handled with grace and maybe a laugh or two. So, let's see what we need to master the art of diapering and manage the inevitable mess.

The Options

Navigating the world of diaper options can feel like a bewildering adventure, with choices ranging from cloth to disposable and everything in between. But don't fret - finding the right fit for your baby and lifestyle is totally doable. Whether you're looking for eco-friendly alternatives, budget-friendly picks, or just the easiest option for those late-night changes, there's a diaper out there for you. Let's take a quick look at what we've got.

- **Disposable Diapers.** These are popular for their convenience - use them, toss them, and you're done. They're perfect for those middle-of-the-night changes when your brain is on autopilot. However, they can be pricey and aren't the best for the environment.

- **Cloth diapers.** They're reusable, eco-friendly, and can save you money in the long run. But they require a bit more effort, as you'll need to wash them regularly.

- **Eco-friendly Disposable Diapers.** If you're looking for a middle ground, then these might be your answer. Made from sustainable materials, they offer guilt-free convenience.

Whatever option you go for, don't forget to stock up because you'll be changing diapers more often than you check your phone. And crucially, remember to choose the right diaper size. A snug fit prevents leaks, but too tight, and your baby will be uncomfortable.

The Diaper Changing Guide

Changing diapers might seem like a daunting task at first, but with a bit of practice and a lot of patience, you'll have it down in no time. From choosing the right supplies to mastering the quick change, this guide's got you covered.

- **Prepare Your Supplies.** Ensure you have all the essentials within arm's reach - clean diapers, wipes, creams, a changing pad and a change of clothes (because, trust me, things can get messy very quickly). For cloth diapers, add a liner and cover.

- **Safety and Hygiene.** Lay your baby on a clean, secure surface, and always keep one hand on them, especially on a raised surface like a changing table.

- **Undo the Dirty Diaper.** Unfasten the dirty diaper and hold your breath if you need to - some of those first ones are next-level. Use the front part to wipe away the bulk of the mess before reaching for the wipes.

- **Clean Up.** Use wipes to clean your baby thoroughly from front to back, especially if they've had a bowel movement. Make sure to get into all those tiny creases.

- **Remove and Dispose of the Dirty Diaper.** Lift your tiny tot's legs and slide the dirty diaper out. To minimise the mess, fold up the dirty diaper, and if it's a disposable one, toss it in the diaper bin, or if it's a cloth diaper, in a wet bag for washing. (You may also want to place dirty diapers in scented bags to help neutralise smelly odours).

- **Slip in the Fresh Diaper.** Slide a clean diaper under your baby's bottom, ensuring it's centred.

- **Secure the Diaper.** Fasten the tabs snugly but not too tight. Ensure the diaper edges are fluffed out to prevent leaks.

Diaper Rash

Let's face it; diaper rash happens! But don't worry; managing it is easier than you think. With a few simple tips and a bit of TLC, you can keep your baby's bottom smooth and happy. From choosing the right products to knowing when to give some extra air time, these tips will help you tackle those pesky rashes with confidence.

- Keep your little one's skin clean and dry, and change diapers frequently.

- Use barrier creams with zinc oxide to protect your baby's sensitive skin.

- Let your baby go diaper-free for short periods to allow their skin to breathe, reducing moisture buildup.

- If a rash does appear, a warm bath and gentle pat dry can soothe irritation. Think of it as a little spa day for your baby's bottom.

Diaper emergencies
These tend to happen when you least expect them. Whether it's a blowout at the worst possible moment or a sudden shortage of diapers, staying calm is key. Always keep a well-stocked diaper bag with essentials like a portable changing mat, extra diapers, plenty of wipes, and a change of clothes for your little one. Quick clean-up solutions, such as travel-sized sanitisers and resealable bags for soiled items, also come in handy. When disaster strikes, a sense of humour goes a long way in diffusing the situation. Roll with the punches, and know that every dad's been there. Remember, these moments will make for great stories down the line.

Okay, diaper duty isn't glamorous, but with a bit of practice and a lot of patience, you'll be able to handle it like a pro. So, keep your sense of humour, stay calm, and embrace the opportunity to bond with your baby. And don't be afraid to ask for help if you need it.

Bathing and Hygiene: Keeping Baby Clean

Bath time is one of those magical moments of the newborn phase. It combines bonding, fun, and cleanliness. Apart from the right gear, you'll also need the two P's - patience and practice. It is essential to keep your tiny tot clean. So, what does it take to keep your baby squeaky clean without turning the bathroom into a waterpark?

What You Need

Bathing your baby can be a fun and soothing experience for both of you, but you'll need a few essentials to make it safe and enjoyable.

- **Baby Bathtub.** A small tub and/or baby bath support will help keep your baby safe and comfy during bath time, reducing the risk of slips and making the whole process much less stressful.

- **Gentle Baby Soap and Shampoo.** Opt for mild, hypoallergenic products designed specifically for babies. They're free from harsh chemicals and fragrances, keeping your little one's skin soft and irritation-free.

- **Bath Thermometer.** This handy tool ensures the water's just the right temperature. Aim for a warm bath, around 37°C (98.6°F), which is just right for your little one's delicate skin. Don't take the water temperature for granted!

- **Soft Washcloths or Flannels.** Use these to gently cleanse your baby without irritating their skin.

- **Towels.** Have a few soft, absorbent towels on hand, preferably with cute hoods to keep your baby warm after their bath.

- **Baby Lotion.** Keep your baby's skin soft and moisturised with gentle, baby-friendly lotion.

- **Diapers and Wipes.** After bath time, make sure you have clean diapers and wipes ready for a fresh start.

- **Clean Clothes.** Have a cosy, clean outfit ready for your baby after their bath to keep them warm and snug.

How to Give Your Baby a Sponge Bath

Some experts say newborns don't need a full bath every day. That, in fact, a gentle sponge bath every few days is just fine until their umbilical cord stump falls off. Here's how you do it:

- **Gather Supplies.** You'll need a bowl of warm water, mild baby soap, soft washcloths and a towel, and make sure they're all within arm's reach so you're not scrambling around mid-bath.

- **Safety First.** From my little experience, bathing your little one can sometimes feel like handling a slippery fish. So, always keep one hand on your baby.

- **Start with the Face.** Use a damp washcloth (no soap) to gently clean your baby's face. Pay extra attention to the neck folds - milk tends to hide there.

- **Move to the Body.** Add a tiny bit of mild baby soap to the washcloth and gently clean your baby's body. Be sure to get into all those cute creases and folds.

- **Rinse and Dry.** Use a damp, clean washcloth to rinse off the soap and a soft towel to pat your baby dry, ensuring they're nice and cosy.

When and How to Transition to a Tub Bath

Once the umbilical cord stump is gone, it's showtime. You can transition to tub baths. This is how we do it:

- **Fill the Tub.** Use a baby bathtub with, where possible, baby bath support. Fill the tub with a few inches of warm water (around 37°C/98.6°F).

- **Support and Safety.** Gently lower your baby into the water, supporting their head and neck. A gentle, firm grip ensures they feel secure – remember, they're still slippery! Use one hand to support them while the other hand washes. Safety is paramount, so never leave your baby unattended, even for a second.

- **The Wash.** Start with your baby's face and work your way down, using a soft cloth or your hand.

- **Rinse, Gentle and Quick.** Keep the bath brief (5-10 minutes). Use your hand or a cup to pour water gently over their body, keeping them warm.

- **Pat Dry and Cuddle.** Once clean, use a soft, warm towel to pat your baby dry, paying special attention to the creases where moisture can linger. Wrap them up and enjoy some cosy cuddle time.

- **It's a Wrap.** Wrap them up and enjoy some cosy cuddle time.

Not Water Friendly
It's easy to assume that babies love water, but that's not always the case. When your baby isn't a water fan, bathing can be a daunting experience. So, to spice things up a little and make the bathing experience a fun adventure, try introducing bath toys. You'd be surprised at what a rubber ducky could do. Then, as they become more comfortable in the water, you can gradually increase their bath time.

Beyond the Bath

Picture a tiny salon session with an unpredictable client who's more interested in exploring their toes than getting a makeover. Welcome to the world of baby grooming. So, what's this about? I hear you ask.

- **Nail Care.** Baby nails grow surprisingly fast, and those tiny daggers can leave scratches. Use a file or baby nail clippers to keep them in check. You could compare trimming your baby's nails to a delicate operation. So, it's best done while the baby is sleeping or very calm to avoid any sudden movements.

- **Hair Care.** Depending on whether your baby has a few wisps or a full head of hair, gentle brushing can help keep things tidy. Using a soft-bristled brush or a baby comb is ideal. Be warned, this may involve a bit of distraction, a lot of cooing, and possibly a dance routine to keep your little one entertained.

- **Ear Cleaning.** Gently clean your baby's outer ear with a damp cloth. Avoid inserting anything into the baby's ear canal. A word of advice: To keep baby's ears healthy and free from wax buildup, you might have to do this regularly.

- **Skin Care.** And, of course, how could we forget the post-bath soothing massage. The gentle application of baby lotion keeps your baby's skin soft and prevents dryness. A light massage can also be a relaxing bonding experience.

- **Cradle Cap.** There's a high possibility that your little one might get this, but there's no need to worry. So, what is cradle cap? Well, it's said to be a harmless skin condition that shows up as scaly patches on a baby's scalp, face, or diaper area. Though it sounds scary and looks unsightly, the good news is it can easily be managed in various ways, such as using a gentle baby brush, applying some baby oil, and using steroid creams, just to mention a few. However, if your baby gets really uncomfortable or you find yourself getting very concerned, don't hesitate to pay your doctor a visit.

Remember, bath time isn't just about cleanliness; it's about creating a relaxing and enjoyable experience for your baby. Keep it gentle and safe, and enjoy the giggles and splashes. Sing a song, talk to them, and cherish these precious moments together; you'll both come out of it feeling refreshed and closer than ever.

Soothing Techniques: Calming a Fussy Baby

Ah, the sweet sound of a baby's cry - not quite music to your ears, but definitely a catchy tune that will be on repeat for a while. Understanding why babies cry is like cracking a code. Often, it boils down to a few usual suspects:

- **Hunger.** Is your baby sucking on their fist or smacking their lips? That's the universal sign for "Feed me, please!"

- **Tiredness.** From yawns and eye-rubbing to drooping eyelids and zoning out, babies have their own ways of saying, "I'm ready for some shut-eye!"

- **Overstimulation.** Fussiness, turning their head away, sudden crying spells or even too much excitement can turn a happy baby into a cranky one.

- **Pain and Discomfort.** From sudden shrill, piercing crying fits and grimacing to pulling their legs up or arching their back, these signals can clue you in when your little one is feeling uncomfortable or in pain.

Once you've figured out the why, it's time to tackle the how.

Here are a few things you can do to calm your fussy baby:

- **Swaddling.** This is a time-tested technique that can work wonders. A snug wrap mimics the snugness of the womb, providing comfort and security.

- **Rocking.** Gentle rocking or slow swaying motions can work wonders. You could also try a rocking chair or even walking while holding them. This has been found to be a valuable recipe for calm.

- **White Noise.** This can be a miracle worker. Soft sounds like a fan, a white noise machine, or even shushing can be incredibly soothing, drowning out other noises and recreating the muffled sounds of the womb. And if music is your thing, you can go for gentle lullabies or soft classical tunes.

- **A Scenery Change.** You never know, but A quick stroll around the house or outside can distract and calm a fussy baby. This definitely worked for my daughters.

- **A Calming Environment.** This is all about setting the stage for relaxation. Dimming the lights can signal bedtime, and reducing noise helps soothe frazzled nerves. Consistency is key – you can ease the transition from playtime to sleep by establishing a bedtime routine.

- **The Mighty Pacifier.** I know some parents aren't exactly great fans of this, but sometimes, a good suck on a pacifier can bring instant calm.

- **The Usual Suspects.** This can sometimes be overlooked, but make sure your baby has been fed, has a clean diaper, and isn't too hot or cold.

- **And If All Those Don't Work.** Of course, even the best

plans can go awry, and sometimes, your baby's fussiness may seem inexplicable. Persistent crying, especially if accompanied by other symptoms, might warrant a visit to the paediatrician. Trust your instincts; if something feels off, it's better to seek reassurance from a professional. They can check for underlying issues and provide peace of mind. Remember, you're not alone in this. Seeking help is not a sign of weakness; it's a strength.

Over time, you'll find your rhythm and learn what works best for you and your baby. With patience and perseverance, these moments of fussiness will become opportunities for bonding and understanding.

Bath time's here, it's splashy and fun,
Rub-a-dub-dub, clean when done.
Diaper duty, you're ever ready,
Quick with the wipes, hold baby steady.

Baby cues, time to decipher the code,
Hungry, sleepy, or just in playful mode?
From burps to coos, you're in the groove,
Ever-ready with the perfect move.

You're in the flow; you've tied it down
You've won your baby's bootcamp crown
With love and care and playful cheer,
You're a star, your little one's pioneer!

~ akin.o ~

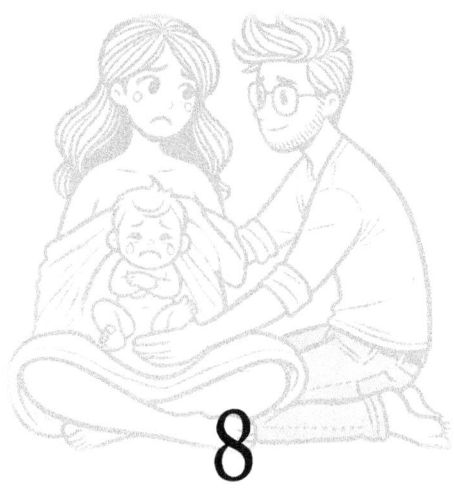

8

The Fourth Trimester
Navigating Postpartum

So, you and your partner have made it through pregnancy and delivery. Thank God! Baby's home and you're just about running on autopilot. But now comes a phase so often overlooked: The Fourth Trimester. It's a transformative time not just for your baby but for your partner and you as well. While your baby is getting acquainted with the world outside the womb, your partner is navigating the complex aftermath of childbirth. It's a period filled with significant physical and emotional changes, and understanding these shifts can make all the difference.

Post-Childbirth Reality Check

After the excitement of childbirth, your partner's body goes into recovery mode. Whether she had a vaginal birth or a C-section, her body has been through a lot. But recovery is so much more than just physical healing; it's also about adjusting to new realities.

- For vaginal births, she might experience lochia, a type of discharge that can last for several weeks and is perfectly normal. If she had a C-section, keeping the incision clean and dry is crucial to avoid infection.

- Hormonal shifts are another factor, often causing fatigue and mood swings that can seem like a never-ending rollercoaster.

- Breastfeeding, despite its benefits, comes with its own set of challenges. Engorgement, or the swelling of the breasts, can be uncomfortable, but frequent feeding and warm compresses can offer relief.

Navigating the Baby Blues

Then there's the emotional and psychological landscape to navigate.

- The baby blues can feel like an unexpected emotional storm after giving birth. Your partner might find herself feeling extra weepy, irritable, or just overwhelmed for no apparent reason. I've heard new mothers say that it's as if their hormones simply decided to take on a mind of their own. Though the baby blues are common, the good news is that it usually passes within a couple of weeks.

- However, if these feelings persist or worsen, they might indicate postpartum depression (PPD). Signs of PPD include overwhelming sadness, anxiety, and a lack of interest in the baby. Recognising these signs early is key to getting the necessary support. This is where your role becomes vital. By actively listening and offering empathetic support, you can help her feel less isolated and more understood. Simple acts like sitting together for a cup of tea and letting her express herself without judgment can be incredibly healing.

Lightening the Postpartum Load

Your practical support can help lighten the load on your

partner, making daily life more manageable as she recovers.

- **Household Chores.** Consider taking charge of household chores and errands. It might seem like a small gesture, but vacuuming the house or tackling a pile of laundry can significantly ease her burden.

- **Meal Prep.** This is another area where you can step in. Planning and preparing meals ensures your partner's getting the nutrition she needs. It's also one less thing for her to worry about.

- **Night Feeds.** Helping out with night-time feeds and diaper changes also helps lighten the load on your partner. Apart from giving her a chance to rest, it also allows you to bond with your baby.

- **Attending Appointments Together.** Don't overlook the importance of scheduling and attending paediatric appointments together. It's a chance to ask questions and stay informed about your baby's health.

Heart-to-Heart

Open communication is the lifeline that keeps your relationship strong during this recovery phase.

- **Daily Check-Ins.** Setting aside daily check-in times can make a world of difference. These moments allow both of you to share your thoughts and feelings and will help foster a deeper connection.

- **A Safe Space.** Creating a safe space where both of you can be honest and vulnerable is invaluable. Encourage your partner to express herself freely, without fear of judgment. By understanding her needs and offering your support, you reinforce the partnership that will carry you through this challenging yet rewarding phase.

Stronger Together

Lastly, remember that you don't have to do it all alone. External support can be a game-changer. Whether it's trusted family and friends or professional services, reaching out for help can lighten the load and provide much-needed respite.

- Family members might be eager to lend a hand, whether it's babysitting for a couple of hours or swinging by with a home-cooked meal. Every little helps!

- Professional services, such as postpartum doulas - your personal baby whisperers and sanity savers all rolled into one, ready with tips and tricks to help you and your partner navigate the maze of newborn life - or cleaning services, can offer additional support tailored to your needs.

Embracing this help doesn't make you less capable; it makes you resourceful, ensuring your family thrives during this transition.

Balancing Support and Personal Well-being

As a new dad, it's so easy to get carried away with looking after the little one that we forget we're also meant to encourage our partner's self-care and our personal well-being. Getting the balance right is essential for maintaining a happy, healthy family dynamic.

Her Much-Needed R&R

Encouraging your partner to take time out to enjoy little luxuries is crucial. You could:

- **A Luxury Soak.** Set her up with a luxurious, long, hot bath where she can soak away the day's stress and emerge feeling like a new person. Think candles, bubbles, and a playlist of her favourite tunes.

- **Pampering Sessions.** Arrange pampering sessions for your beloved partner. Whether it's a home spa day or a professional massage, this is one luxury that's essential for her recovery.

- **Relaxation Time.** Schedule some all-important solo relaxation time for her when you can take over baby duties. A nap or a quiet moment with a book can work wonders.

- **Regular Breaks.** Encourage her to take regular breaks. You'd be surprised at what 10 minutes of alone time can do.

- **Childcare Swaps.** Organise childcare swaps, but only with trusted friends or family, and only if that's your thing. Trading babysitting duties can give your partner a chance to recharge while strengthening your support network.

Knowing she's got these moments to herself can make the demands of parenthood a bit more manageable.

Stay Balanced and Energised

Meanwhile, don't forget about yourself. Your well-being is just as important, and maintaining it will help you be there for your family. Here are a few things you can do to keep your well-being batteries charged:

- **Keep Moving!.** Regular physical activity, even if it's just a walk around the block or a few push-ups in the living room, can do wonders. You'd be amazed at what a little movement can do for your mood and energy.

- **Hobbies.** Take time for your hobbies and interests. Whether it's writing lyrics, tinkering with a car, or going out for a game of badminton, doing something you love will keep you grounded.

- **A Balanced Diet.** Make sure you're eating a balanced diet that's rich in nutrients. Remember, a healthy body leads to a healthy mind.

- **Personal Breaks.** While you're encouraging your partner to take regular breaks, don't forget to take them yourself. Even a short one can help you recharge and stay focused.

- **Catch a Nap.** And don't forget to catch as much sleep as you can. Naps can be Dad's best friend during these times, so grab them whenever possible.

Remember, it's impossible to pour from an empty cup, so keep fit, nourished and well-rested, ready for the long nights ahead.

Syncing Parenthood and Personal Time

Balancing the responsibilities of new parenthood with personal needs requires a bit of strategy. Here are a few things that can help:

- **Shared Calendars.** Creating a shared calendar can be a game-changer. You can use it to map out household duties, childcare, and even downtime. This visual aid helps distribute tasks evenly so no one feels overloaded.

- **Leisure Time.** Negotiating leisure time for individual and joint activities is also essential. Maybe you both enjoy watching a good movie or cooking together. Make it a priority to carve out time for these shared experiences, as well as individual pursuits.

- **Be Flexible.** Parenting requires flexibility, so stay flexible. Adjust your plans as needed to ensure you're taking care of yourself while managing parental duties.

Making time for regular breaks and those much-loved hobbies is also essential. In a nutshell, it's all about finding that sweet spot where responsibilities and relaxation coexist.

Boundaries and Balance: Beating Burnout
Finding the right balance as a new parent can sometimes feel like walking a tightrope. And because you've got a million things to juggle, it's all too easy to lose sight of your own well-being. So, here are some practical tips and tricks to help you keep the scales tipped in your favour.

- **You Can Say "No!".** Don't hesitate to say "no" if you're feeling overwhelmed. It's okay to limit commitments and focus on what truly matters. Trust your instincts and know when to step back.

- **Manageable Goals.** Set small, manageable goals each day, like folding a load of laundry or prepping a meal. These bite-sized tasks are achievable and prevent the sense of being buried under a mountain of chores. By keeping expectations reasonable, you create a sustainable routine that nurtures both your family and yourself.

- **Recognise Burnout Signs.** Now, this is crucial. If you notice persistent fatigue, irritability, or a lack of joy in activities once enjoyed, it might be time to reassess. These symptoms can creep up slowly, like a fog rolling in.

- **Seek Professional Support if Needed.** Therapy or counselling can offer guidance and coping strategies, ensuring you maintain your mental health. I'll say this again, "Asking for help is a strength, not a weakness".

- **Prioritise Self-Care.** Remember, taking care of yourself benefits your entire family.

Here's the deal. Setting boundaries and finding balance is key to beating burnout. Pace yourself, prioritise self-care, and keep yourself healthy and happy. That's the best way to be there for your little one and family without losing your sanity.

Keeping the Romance Alive

It's easy for romance to take a back seat when you're knee-deep in the chaos of diaper changes and midnight feeds. But don't worry – it's totally doable and can be a lot of fun. It's the small things that tend to reignite that spark, those little moments and gestures that show you care. So, let's look at some simple yet effective ways to keep that romantic flame burning bright.

- **Date Nights.** Arranging regular date nights at home or out can be a game-changer. It doesn't have to be anything extravagant. A quiet dinner at your favourite local spot can remind you both of the connection that brought you together. For those evenings when leaving the house feels like a Herculean task, get creative with at-home date nights. You could transform your living room into a romantic haven for a cosy home movie night or pick a dish both of you have never tried before and turn the kitchen into your own culinary adventure. Once you settle into a routine, planning weekend getaways can offer a much-needed escape, allowing you to recharge and reconnect without the usual distractions.

- **Surprise Gestures.** Little surprise gestures, like writing a heartfelt note or getting her favourite treat, can do wonders for your relationship. These unexpected acts of kindness and thoughtfulness remind her that she's cherished and appreciated and keeps the magic alive in the everyday hustle and bustle.

- **Shared Hobbies.** Engaging in activities you both like and having fun together is like adding a double scoop of joy to your relationship sundae. Whether cooking up a storm together, hitting the hiking trails, getting competitive with board games or enjoying a shared hobby, these activities create memorable moments and strengthen your bond. It's about laughing over a failed recipe, celebrating little victories, and enjoying each other's company.

- **Open communication.** This is like the magic glue that keeps a relationship strong and vibrant. It's all about sharing your thoughts, dreams, and even the silly things that make you laugh. Imagine a walk in the park, sitting down over a cuppa, just talking about your day, your hopes, or even that weird dream you had last night. It's a sure way to connect, both emotionally and physically. Being honest and open creates a deeper connection and understanding between you and your partner. Plus, it's a great way to avoid misunderstandings and keep the love flowing smoothly.

- **Celebrate the Small Moments.** Amidst all the chaos, it's vital to celebrate the small moments of joy and achievement together. Did you manage to get the baby to sleep before midnight? Celebrate it! Did you both survive a week of work and parenting duties? High-fives all around! Recognising and acknowledging these small victories can bring you closer, reinforcing your partnership and reminding you of the love that underpins everything else. It's these little moments of shared laughter and triumph that weave the fabric of your relationship, making it resilient and strong.

- **Physical affection.** This is the key to maintaining intimacy. A warm hug after a long day, a gentle kiss on the forehead, or just holding hands while watching TV are little gestures that speak volumes. They say, "I'm here for you," without uttering a word. Plus, they release those feel-good hormones that make everything seem a bit brighter. So, don't shy away from those cuddles and kisses – they're the secret sauce that keeps the love sizzling in a relationship!

In the whirlwind of dadhood, keeping the romance alive requires effort and intention. You and your Mrs need to carve out moments just for the two of you, and with a sprinkle of creativity, you can nurture the connection that brought you together in the first place. Remember, it's about cherishing the small things and finding joy in each other's presence, even amidst the chaos of midnight feeds and sleepless nights.

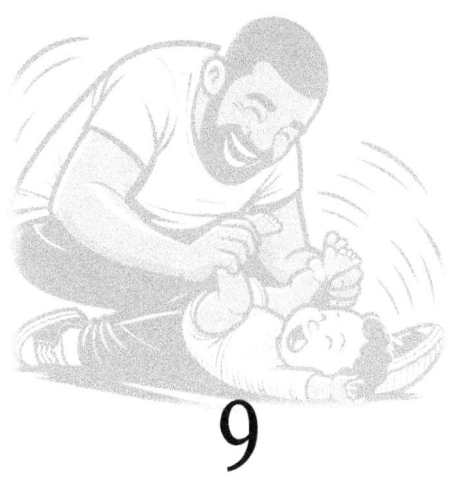

9

The Bonding
Dad and Baby Time

As you've heard me mention before, becoming a dad is like stepping onto a rollercoaster - exciting, a bit scary, and loads of ups and downs. At the core of this wild ride is the bond you build with your baby. It's the glue that holds everything together. Whether it's late-night feeds and diaper changes, silly face contests, or those quiet moments of snuggling, every interaction is a chance to connect. As a first-time dad, building a strong bond with your baby is one of the most important and rewarding things you'll do, and it starts from day one. But how do you foster this bond?

Kangaroo Care Moments

A practice as old as time yet revolutionary in its simplicity, kangaroo care is a match made in parenting heaven! Still One of the most effective ways to bond with your baby, this magical ritual involves skin-to-skin contact, where you hold your little one against your bare chest. According to the experts, when you do this, your body releases oxytocin, often called the "love hormone." This hormone creates feelings of warmth and attachment. For your baby, this bonding process helps regulate their temperature and heartbeat while boosting their immune system and promoting emotional well-being. It makes your tiny tot feel like they're back in the womb but with a much better view. It's not just cute - it's crucial for their development. And as a dad, you get to experience that magical feeling of connecting with your baby on a deeper level. So, what can you do to enhance this practice?

Create a Cosy Bonding Oasis
To get started, create a cosy environment. Think of it as setting the stage for a peaceful bonding session. Choose a quiet, warm room where distractions are minimal. A soft blanket draped over your shoulder can provide extra warmth, but ensure your baby is only wearing a diaper to maximise skin-to-skin contact. Gently lay your baby on your chest, positioning them so their ear is over your heart. This familiar sound will soothe and calm them. Support their head and neck with one hand, allowing your other arm to wrap securely around their body. It's a moment of stillness where the outside world fades away, and it's just you and your baby.

A Daily Routine
Incorporating skin-to-skin into your daily routine is easier than you might think. Post-bath cuddles are a perfect opportunity. Once your little one is squeaky clean, wrap them in a towel and snuggle up for some skin-to-skin warmth. Bedtime routines and morning bonding sessions can also be transformed with this practice. Start or end your day with a few minutes of peaceful contact, helping your baby feel safe and loved while reinforcing your bond. It's a gentle reminder that amidst the chaos of diapers and midnight feedings, these quiet moments are what truly matter.

Snuggles Amidst the Hustle

Of course, life gets busy, and finding time for skin-to-skin can seem like a challenge. Juggling work schedules might make it feel like there's never enough time. But even a few minutes can make a difference, so don't stress about the clock. Fit it in where you can, perhaps during a lunch break or before you leave for work. You might also feel self-conscious. It's natural to feel a bit awkward at first, especially if you're new to this. But remember, your baby doesn't care about your dad bod or your questionable choice of music as long as they can hear your heartbeat and feel your warmth. Embrace this opportunity to connect and let go of any insecurities.

Babywearing

This is all about carrying your baby close to your body using a wrap, sling, or carrier while you have both hands free to conquer your day. Think of yourself as a human kangaroo. This makes grocery shopping, strolls in the park, and household chores a breeze. But this isn't just about convenience; it's also perfect for bonding! By keeping your baby nestled snugly against your chest, happily gurgling away, you're offering them a front-row seat to the world, all from the comfort of your embrace. This closeness fosters a deep emotional connection, helping your baby feel secure and loved. As you move, your baby's senses are engaged, supporting their physical development through the gentle sway and rhythm of your steps. It's like giving them a dance lesson while you go about your day.

Finding the Perfect Fit

Choosing the right baby carrier can feel like navigating a maze, but with a few pointers, you'll find the perfect match. Consider the various types:

- **Wrap Carriers.** These are versatile and snug, perfect for newborns who love that close, womb-like feel.

- **Slings Carriers.** This offers a simple, over-the-shoulder option that is ideal for quick trips.

- **Structured Carriers.** As these come with ergonomic support, they are great for longer adventures and growing babies.

Each carrier type has its perks. What's important is that you think about your lifestyle and comfort preferences when making your choice. Personally, I believe ergonomic design is key. So, I would advise you to go for a carrier offering adequate support for you and your baby.

Tips for Babywearing Bliss

Safety is paramount in babywearing. Here are a few guidelines to help ensure a positive experience:

- Always check for proper positioning, ensuring your baby's head and neck are well-supported.

- Keep their airways clear, with their chin off their chest, and ensure their hips are in a healthy position. A good rule of thumb is to keep them high enough on your chest that you can easily kiss the top of their head.

- Regularly check the carrier's fit and make adjustments as needed.

- Your comfort matters, too, so distribute the weight evenly to avoid straining your back.

Making Babywearing a Lifestyle

Incorporating babywearing into daily life is a breeze, and you'll wonder how you ever managed without it.

- Take leisurely walks in the park, letting your baby enjoy the sights and sounds of nature right alongside you.

- Need to tackle household chores? Strap on your carrier and get to work - your baby will love being part of the action. Whether you're vacuuming or folding laundry, they'll feel like they're helping out.

- And, of course, it's also perfect for social events and gatherings, keeping your baby close while you catch up with friends. Just remember, with your baby snug against you, you'll be the centre of attention, and that's a beautiful thing.

Stimulating Your Baby's Development

When it comes to your baby's world, play isn't just a way to pass the time – it's a crucial part of their cognitive and emotional growth. Play is how they learn to make sense of the world around them. It's like a secret language, one you both get to learn together. As a dad, you're not just a spectator in this vibrant world; you're the co-pilot, guiding your little one through the wonders of sensory exploration and motor skill development. Imagine your baby's delight as they discover the feel of different textures or the joy of cause and effect when they shake a rattle. Each playful moment is a building block, fostering their understanding of shapes, sounds, and colours. Your role is to be right there with them, encouraging this exploration and cheering on every tiny victory.

Crafting the Perfect Play Haven
Creating a play-conducive environment at home is like setting the stage for a grand performance. Start by selecting age-appropriate toys and materials, ensuring they're safe and stimulating. A clean, hazard-free play zone is paramount. Think of it as their personal playground, where

imagination runs wild and creativity has no boundaries. Clear away potential hazards, ensure the space is inviting and comfortable, and maybe add a soft rug for some tummy time. Remember, this is your baby's domain, and your job is to make it as inviting and exciting as possible.

Building Skills Through Fun
Age-appropriate play activities are your tools of the trade. For the littlest ones, tummy time is where it's at. While it might look like they're just chilling on their belly, they're actually working hard, strengthening those little muscles and preparing for crawling. As they grow, games like peek-a-boo can become a go-to activity. It's not just about the giggles; it's about engaging their visual tracking and social skills. Soft toys and rattles provide tactile stimulation, allowing them to explore through touch and sound. These toys are more than just playthings; they're instruments for development, sparking curiosity and joy.

Harmonising Playtime Structure and Creativity
Balancing structured and unstructured play can be like cooking the perfect meal - each ingredient adds something special. Guided activities with specific goals can help your little one learn new skills, like stacking blocks or sorting shapes. These activities provide structure and direction, offering opportunities for learning and growth. On the flip side, unstructured play is all about creativity and self-expression. Letting them explore freely encourages imagination and problem-solving. It's the difference between following a recipe and creating a dish from scratch. Both have their place and together, they create a rich tapestry of play that nourishes your baby's development.

Creative Bonding Activities

It's been a long day, and you're sitting with your baby in the soft glow of a nightlight, crooning a lullaby. It's a moment of pure magic, but did you know it's also a powerful tool for development? Singing and storytelling aren't just for keeping babies entertained; they play a crucial role in language growth and emotional bonding. As you sing, those repetitive lyrics aren't just catchy; they're expanding your baby's vocabulary. Every "Twinkle, Twinkle" is a building block for their future communication. And when you weave a story, you're not just telling a tale - you're creating emotional connections. Through characters and plots, your baby learns about emotions, empathy, and the comfort of your voice.

Pick the Perfect Bedtime Playlist
Choosing the right songs and stories is like crafting the perfect playlist. You want a mix that resonates with your baby and sets them up for sweet dreams. Classic lullabies and nursery rhymes are timeless for a reason - they're simple, rhythmic, and easy for little ones to follow. Think "Rock-a-bye Baby" or "Mary Had a Little Lamb." These tunes are the perfect bedtime companions. For storytime, board books with vivid illustrations and simple narratives are key. Titles like "Goodnight Moon" or "The Very Hungry Caterpillar" captivate with their bright colours and engaging tales. They're not just books but gateways into a world of imagination and wonder.

Add Melody Moments to Everyday Routines
Incorporating music and stories into your daily routine doesn't require a grand production - just a little creativity, like singing during diaper changes or bath time. This transforms mundane tasks into moments of joy and engagement. Let your voice fill the room with playful melodies. Establishing a bedtime story ritual signals winding down, creating a calming atmosphere for sleep. Your soothing voice is the soundtrack to their dreams, providing consistency and comfort. This routine becomes a cherished part of your day, a signal that it's time to relax and unwind.

Creative Stories with a Personal Twist

Creating personalised stories and songs is your chance to channel your inner bard. Use family members and pets as characters, turning your baby's world into a personal fairy tale. Imagine a story where their favourite stuffed animal goes on an adventure or a song with their name woven into the chorus. This isn't just about being creative; it's about making memories that are uniquely yours. These tales become a part of your family culture, a shared history that your child will treasure as they grow.

Baby Cues: The Must Learn Language

Your baby might not have a complete vocabulary yet, but they're constantly communicating with you through their cues. You'd be surprised at how communicative your little one is, even without a single syllable. Understanding your baby's cues is like learning a new language - one that involves more yawns and grunts than words. So, as a first-time dad, how do you recognise, understand and decode this new baby language?

- **Crying.** This is your baby's primary way of communicating, and believe it or not, there are different cry types. It can be tricky to figure out what each cry means, but with time, you'll start recognising them. There's the hungry cry, the tired cry, the uncomfortable cry, and, of course, the "I just want a cuddle" cry. When your baby cries, do your best to respond quickly and lovingly. This teaches them that they can trust you to meet their needs.

- **Facial Expressions.** Your baby's face is a treasure trove of emotions. Those tiny eyebrows, the wide-eyed wonder, and the little frowns are all clues to how your baby is feeling. Pay attention to their facial expressions and respond with your own. Smile back when they smile, and comfort them when they look worried. This mirroring helps to strengthen your bond.

- **Body Language.** Your little one also communicates through their body language. Turning their head toward anything that brushes their cheek (referred to as "rooting") and sucking on their hands are common hunger cues. It's as if they're saying, "Feed me, please!" Then there's the yawn, the universal symbol of tiredness. Rubbing eyes and appearing glazed over are also dead giveaways that it's time for a nap. The discomfort cues, such as arching their back or a sharp grunt, might indicate gas or an awkward position. When you tune in to these cues, you can respond more effectively to your baby's needs.

- **Coos and Gurgles.** As your baby grows, they'll start to make all sorts of delightful sounds - coos, gurgles, and giggles. These sounds are their way of interacting with you and the world around them. Engage with these sounds by talking back, mimicking their noises, and making silly faces. This back-and-forth interaction is a crucial part of bonding and language development.

- **The Power of Eye Contact.** Never underestimate the power of eye contact. When your baby looks into your eyes, they're not just staring - they're learning and connecting. Take the time to look into their eyes during feedings, diaper changes, and playtime. It's these little moments that build trust and love.

- **Words Matter.** This one's more on you than a baby cue. Though your baby might not understand your words, they sure do understand your tone. Talking to your baby in a soothing, calm voice can help them feel secure. Narrate your day, sing songs, or just chat about anything. It's not about what you say - it's the connection you're building through your voice.

- **Pattern Mapping.** Here's another one that's on you. Tracking and learning patterns in your baby's cues can be a game-changer. Keep a notebook or use an app to log interactions and identify patterns. Jot down what cues lead to what needs, and over time, you'll start to see a pattern. Reflect on what works and what doesn't, adjusting your strategies as needed. It's like creating a personalised guide for your baby that evolves as they do. Understanding these patterns lets you become more intuitive, turning guesswork into insight.

If you're like me, there will be times when you'll feel like a detective, piecing together clues trying to solve the mystery of what your little one needs, but as you become fluent in your baby's unique language, you'll find yourself more connected and confident in your role. Remember, these moments of understanding and responsiveness are the building blocks of a lifelong, loving relationship, setting the stage for an incredible dadhood journey.

The Key is in the Two P's

Bonding with your newborn isn't going to happen overnight; I guess you knew this already. It's a gradual process that requires the dynamic duo - patience and persistence. Patience means being there, ready to catch those fleeting moments of connection, whether it's during a midnight feed or a lazy Sunday cuddle. Persistence is about showing up, day in and day out, building trust and love through consistency. Giving your little one the time they need to connect while staying committed through the ups and downs is a tried and tested bonding formula that won't let you down. There will be times when you'll feel like you're not getting it right or when you're low on confidence, exhausted and frustrated. That's okay. Sticking with it and embracing the journey is what makes those dad moments so special and rewarding. Remember that every small connecting moment adds up. Trust your instincts, stay calm and determined, and be kind to yourself. So, enjoy every step of this incredible adventure, and know you're doing an amazing job.

Cherish Every Moment

There's something undeniably special about dad and baby time. It's a time when the world narrows down to just the two of you, creating memories and building an unbreakable bond. It may be a journey filled with love, laughter, and sleepless nights, but every moment is worth it. So, embrace the chaos, soak in the snuggles, and cherish these early days. They'll go by faster than you can imagine, and once they're gone, you can't get them back!

With bedtime stories and ticklish toes,
Bonding grows deeper, and love overflows.
Sleepless nights and early morning grins,
In your embrace, a new life begins.

Giggles and cuddles, naps in the chair,
This little one knows you're always there.
A bond like no other, unbreakable and true,
Just look at that smile - Dad, it's all for you!

~ akin.o ~

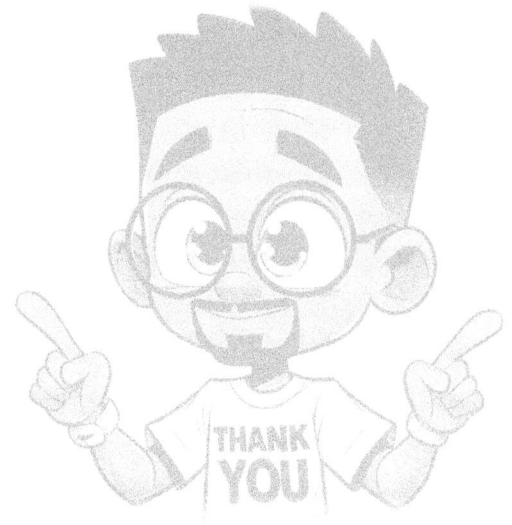

Sharing the Dad Love
Make a Difference with Your Review

"Being a dad isn't about being perfect. It's about being there." ~ *anon*

When I became a dad, there were times when I felt like I'd been handed a unique gadget without any instructions - excited, bewildered, and maybe a little terrified. That's why I poured my heart into writing this guide; to make your ride smoother by helping you navigate this adventure with confidence, humour, and a lot less stress.

Imagine a fellow dad standing in the baby aisle, looking lost and flustered, or holding a diaper in the wee hours of the morning, wondering what to do with it. That dad could use this book. By sharing your story, you can pass on some wisdom and laughter and also give a little nudge of confidence.

Leaving a review for *"The Essential Guide for First-Time Dads"* is quick, free, and easier than assembling a crib (I promise). And, it's impact? HUGE! Your words could…

…bring laughter during anxious times.

...Encourage a partner to feel supported and heard.
...help tackle the early days with confidence.
...and most importantly, be the reassuring whisper saying, "You've got this, Dad!"

It only takes a minute or two to leave a review. Simply scan the QR code and watch your words spark a lifetime of better dadhood moments.

Thanks a ton for being part of this incredible dadhood community and for making it stronger, one review at a time.

Your biggest fan,
akin olunloyo

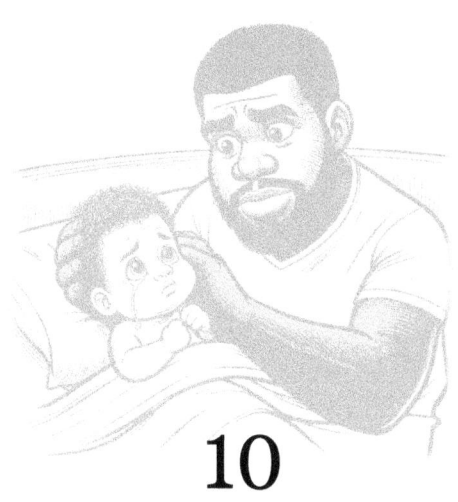

10

Health and Happiness
The Baby Edition

So, there you are on the couch, watching your newborn sleep peacefully in their cot. You're filled with love, awe, and maybe a hint of terror because suddenly, you're not just the cool guy who can change a diaper with one hand; you're also responsible for keeping this tiny human safe and healthy. As a first-time dad, ensuring your baby's health and safety might feel like navigating a minefield of potential hazards and worries. But fear not! With a little know-how and a lot of love, you'll be well-equipped to keep your little one safe and sound. So, welcome to the world of mastering health and safety - a realm where understanding your baby's vital signs is as crucial as creating a safe haven for them. So, let's start with the health side of things.

Understanding Your Baby's Vital Signs

Now, no one expects you to have a medical degree or a stethoscope around your neck, but having a basic grasp of your little one's vitals can make a world of difference. Knowing what's normal and when to call in the pros can give you peace of mind and help ensure your baby is thriving. So, let's break it down into easy-to-digest bits so you can confidently keep tabs on your baby's health and well-being.

- **Temperature.** The normal temperature for your newborn is between 36.5°C (97.7°F) and 37.5°C (99.5°F). Anything above or below might warrant a chat with your paediatrician.

- **Breathing.** This is another critical sign. Your baby is unique and will most likely have an irregular breathing pattern, with pauses lasting up to 10 seconds. It's like they're experimenting with their new lungs. However, if they're consistently breathing rapidly or making grunting sounds, then it's time to knock on your doctor's door.

- **Heartbeat.** It's normal for your newborn's heart rate to be relatively fast, typically between 120-160 beats per minute. If it's consistently too slow or too fast, you know what to do: Hello Doctor!

- **Diaper Counts.** Monitoring wet and dirty diapers can give you a clue about hydration and digestion. If you notice a sudden change in the number of wet diapers or a lack of dirty ones, it might be a sign to check in with your paediatrician. Diaper changes are also a great opportunity to quickly monitor your baby's other vital signs like skin colour and overall comfort. So, keep those diaper counts in check, and you'll have one less thing to stress about!

Common Health Issues

Identifying common newborn illnesses is like developing a sixth sense - one that involves less mysticism and more observation. With its tiny body and growing immune system, your unique baby is prone to a handful of common health issues. From those pesky diaper rashes to the sniffles and beyond, knowing what to look for can help ease the stress and ensure your baby stays healthy and happy. So, here are some of the usual suspects you might encounter.

- **The Sneezy Scenarios.** Your baby is like a tiny magnet for germs; sooner or later, they'll catch a cold or flu. Symptoms can include coughing, a runny nose, and sometimes a fever. Keep them hydrated, and maybe use a humidifier to ease congestion and ensure they get plenty of rest. There's no need to worry; your baby will recover faster than you can say "gesundheit!" And yes, prepare to be sneezed on frequently.

- **The Silent Screamers.** Ear infections are common, especially after a cold. If your baby is unusually fussy, tugging at their ear, or has trouble sleeping, it might be an ear infection, and a trip to the doctor is in order - they might need antibiotics. Meanwhile, do all you can to keep your baby comfortable and reassure them that better days (and nights) are ahead.

- **The Not-So-Great Bottom Situation.** Diaper rash is almost a rite of passage. Those red, irritated patches on your baby's bottom are usually caused by wet or dirty diapers left on for too long. To prevent it, change diapers frequently and use a barrier cream. If a rash does appear, let your baby's skin breathe by allowing them to go diaper-free. Think of it as your baby's spa day.

- **The Drool Fest.** Teething is a messy, drooly business. Symptoms include irritability, drooling, and a tendency to chew on anything within reach. Offer teething rings, gentle gum massages, and lots of cuddles. If your baby's really uncomfortable, ask your paediatrician about pain relief options. Remember, those tiny teeth are coming in for a lifetime of chomping adventures.

- **The Slow-Moving Scenario.** If your baby is straining or their poop is hard and dry, they might be constipated. Increase their fluid intake and, if they're on solids, offer high-fibre foods like pureed prunes or pears. If the issue persists, consult your paediatrician. And yes, you'll develop a weirdly keen interest in poop consistency - it's part of the new dad territory.

- **The Bumpy Road.** Your baby has sensitive skin, which means rashes and irritations are pretty common. Whether it's heat rash, eczema, or an allergic reaction, keep the affected area clean and dry. Use hypoallergenic products and dress your baby in soft, breathable fabrics. Skin rashes can be alarming but are often harmless. However, consult your doctor if a rash doesn't improve or seems to bother your baby.

- **Jaundice.** Many newborns develop jaundice, a yellowing of the skin and eyes. It's usually harmless and goes away on its own. No need to panic, but keep an eye out, especially if it spreads or deepens. And if you're concerned, don't hesitate to consult your paediatrician.

- **Reflux.** Spitting up milk after feeding is common in babies. Once again, it's usually harmless. Just keep those burp cloths handy. Hold your baby upright after meals, and don't worry, they'll outgrow it. If it seems excessive or causes discomfort, talk to your doctor.

- **Colic.** This can cause intense crying and fussiness in otherwise healthy babies. It's tough but temporary and usually resolves itself. Soothing techniques like rocking, swaddling, white noise, or a warm bath can help. Just hang in there - this too shall pass!

Health and Happiness

So there you have it - a quick rundown of some common baby health issues and how to tackle them. Remember, it's all part of the dadhood journey, and with a bit of knowledge and a lot of love, you'll navigate these challenges like a pro. Keep an eye out for those symptoms, trust your instincts, and don't hesitate to reach out to your paediatrician when in doubt. Your little one is in good hands - yours!

Your Baby's Immunity and Well-Being

Ensuring your baby's immunity and overall well-being is like fortifying a tiny fortress. It might sound daunting, but it's all about a few simple, consistent steps which, if kept in check, will help your little one grow up strong and healthy.

- **Breastfeeding.** This is like giving your baby a personalised health boost! Breast milk is packed with antibodies and essential nutrients, which help boost your little one's immune system and support their growth. Whether breastfeeding exclusively or supplementing with formula, every drop counts. Now, I know you can't do this yourself, but your role is vital. From fetching snacks and water during late-night feeds to helping with burping and diaper changes, you can be a real lifesaver as you'll soon realise that being actively involved has a way of strengthening the family bond. And, of course, skin-to-skin cuddles are a great way to bond with your baby and give mum a well-deserved break.

- **Vaccinations.** These are like knights in shining armour as they are crucial for protecting your little one's immune system. These shots help protect your baby against serious illnesses and build their immunity. A vaccination schedule for your baby will be provided by your doctor. Make it a priority and always stick to it. From Hepatitis B to measles, vaccines are timed to when your baby's immune system can best handle and benefit from them. See it as the ultimate health security system with fewer passwords to remember. Watching your baby get a shot can be tough, but the benefits far outweigh the momentary discomfort. After the shot, your baby might be fussy or have a low-grade fever. Keep them comfortable with lots of cuddles and maybe a dose of infant acetaminophen, as recommended by your doctor. And hey, a little extra pampering never hurt anyone - think of it as a well-deserved Dad-and-baby bonding session.

- **Doctor Visits.** These are more than just quick check-ups; they're milestones in your baby's growth and development. Your doctor tracks your baby's weight, length, and head circumference to help ensure they're growing at a healthy rate. They'll also check motor skills, reflexes, and overall health. Before you head to each check-up, jot down any questions or concerns you might have, as it's easy to forget them in the moment. Bring a comfort item for your baby, like their favourite blanket or toy, to ease any anxiety. And don't be surprised if your baby turns into a mini-drama queen at the sight of a stethoscope - it happens to the best of us.

- **Healthy Diet.** Feeding your baby a healthy diet is like fuelling a tiny engine for growth and adventure! As your baby starts on solids, focus on giving them a rainbow of fruits and veggies, along with whole grains and lean proteins, to support their development and help build a strong immune system. Remember, introducing a variety of tastes and textures early on can make mealtime fun and set the stage for healthy eating habits. So, get creative with those purees and finger foods - you're laying the foundation for a lifetime of good nutrition!

- **Good Hygiene.** This is like giving your baby a shield against germs and illness! Regular handwashing, especially before meals and after diaper changes, is super important.

Keeping their environment clean, from toys to bedding, helps minimise the risk of infections. Don't forget bath time - it's not only essential for cleanliness but also a fun bonding activity. By keeping things clean and tidy, you're setting up healthy habits that will benefit your baby now and in the long run!

- **Quality Sleep.** Getting plenty of sleep is like hitting the reset button for your baby's health and happiness! Quality sleep is crucial for their growth, brain development, and overall well-being, and it may be a good idea to establish a steady bedtime routine to help your little one wind down and sleep soundly. Whether it's a warm bath, a gentle lullaby, or a cuddly storytime, these little rituals can make a big difference. Well-rested babies are usually happier and healthier, giving you and your partner some much-needed rest too!

- **Outdoor Play.** This is like a breath of fresh air for your baby's well-being! Sunshine and some fresh air can work wonders for their mental and physical development. Whether a stroll in the park or tummy time on a blanket soaking up nature, these moments are priceless. Outdoor play helps build a strong immune system and allows your baby to explore the world. Always remember to use the appropriate sun protection when it's sunny.

If you keep on top of these elements - from breastfeeding and vaccinations to good hygiene and a healthy diet, and don't underestimate the power of sleep and a bit of outdoor play, too - your little one will grow up strong and healthy. Remember, it's the little things you do every day that make a big difference in your baby's health.

First Aid Basics for First-Time Dads

Accidents happen. You'll want to be prepared when those

inevitable bumps and scrapes occur. So, here's your crash course in baby first aid.

- **Baby's First Aid Kit.** Create a well-stocked first aid kit tailored to your newborn. This should include baby-safe bandages, fun band-aids, antiseptic wipes, gauze pads, adhesive tape, a digital thermometer, tweezers, and infant acetaminophen or ibuprofen. Think of it as your baby's health arsenal - ready to tackle any minor mishap.

- **Cardiopulmonary Resuscitation (CPR).** CPR is a skill every parent should know. It's one of those things you hope you never need, but it's priceless in an emergency. If you haven't already, I'd say enrol in an infant CPR class. There are many options available online or through local community centres. It's an excellent investment.

- **Cuts and Bruises.** Babies are learning to navigate their world, which means tumbles and falls are inevitable. When dealing with cuts, clean the wound with mild soap and water, apply an antiseptic, and cover it with a fun band-aid. For bruises, an ice pack wrapped in a cloth works wonders. Remember, your soothing words and comforting hugs are just as important as the first aid itself. Also, a kiss from Dad has magical healing properties.

- **Fevers.** These can be scary, but they're a natural sign that your baby's body is fighting off an infection. If your baby has a fever, keep them hydrated, dress them in light clothing, and use a digital thermometer to monitor their temperature. Infant acetaminophen can help, but always follow the dosage instructions. If the fever persists or if your baby's temperature exceeds 38°C (100.4°F), then it's time to seek medical advice. Remember, staying cool under pressure is key. Your calm and comforting presence can make all the difference.

- **Colds and Coughs.** Just like adults, babies can catch colds.

Dad's first aid for coughs and colds is all about TLC - tender loving care! Keep your little one hydrated with plenty of fluids, and use a cool-mist humidifier to ease stuffy noses. Gentle pats on the back can help with chest congestion. Don't forget to keep them cosy and offer lots of cuddles. Don't hesitate to give your doctor a buzz if the symptoms persist or worsen.

- **Allergies.** Keep an eye out for common symptoms like itchy eyes, sneezing, swelling, trouble breathing, or rashes. Having antihistamines on hand can be a lifesaver for mild reactions - my daughter suffers from occasional bouts of hay fever, so I can totally identify with this! Knowing how to use an epinephrine injector is crucial for severe allergies. Do your best to create an allergy-friendly environment by minimising exposure to allergens. And most importantly, stay calm and reassuring - your little one looks to you for comfort. I know I'm beginning to sound like a broken record, but don't hesitate to seek medical advice if needed.

- **Choking Hazards.** Babies do a lot of exploring with their mouths. This makes choking a real concern. So, keep a watchful eye, especially during mealtimes, to prevent accidents before they happen. Cut food into tiny, manageable pieces and avoid giving your little one hard-to-chew items like nuts or grapes. If your baby does start choking, stay calm. Lay them face down on your forearm and give gentle back blows between their shoulder blades. If the object doesn't come out, turn your baby over and perform chest thrusts. It's always a good idea to brush up on infant CPR - you never know when you'll need it.

- **Call the Doctor.** Not every bump or fever requires a trip to the Emergency Ward, but knowing when to call the doctor is crucial. If your tiny human has a high fever, persistent crying, difficulty breathing, a severe cut, or any other worrying symptoms, pick up the phone. It's always better to be safe than sorry. Your medical professional is there to help, so never feel like you're overreacting. Seeking professional advice is part of being a great parent. Trust your instincts - if something feels off, it's better to get it checked out.

First aid is all about being prepared and staying calm. Whether it's handling coughs and colds or knowing when to call the doctor, you have what it takes to keep your little one safe and sound. Your baby will inevitably have a few bumps along the way, but with your well-stocked first aid kit and some basic knowledge, you'll handle it like a pro. Plus, every scrape is a chance for a superhero dad moment. Remember, every first-time dad learns on the job.

Your Well-Being: Emotional, Physical and Mental

While you're busy being the household superhero, it's easy to forget about your own health and safety. But remember, you can't pour from an empty cup – I've said that before, right? Taking care of yourself is just as important as looking after your little one. From sneaking in some exercise and eating right to managing stress and getting enough sleep, prioritising your well-being is crucial. Here are some practical tips to keep you in tip-top condition.

- **Stress Management.** Dadhood is rewarding, but it's also stressful. Sleepless nights, endless diaper changes, and the pressure to be the best dad can add up. Find healthy ways to manage stress. From exercise to a hobby that lets you unwind, take time out for yourself - it isn't selfish; it's essential! After all, nobody wants a stressed-out dad moping around the house.

- **The Elusive Dream.** Sleep might feel like a long-lost friend, but getting enough rest is a necessity. Nap when the baby naps, and don't be afraid to ask for help from your tribe if and when required. Remember, even superheroes need rest, and right now, you're your baby's Superman.

- **Stay Physically Active.** Exercise isn't just about avoiding the stereotypical dad bod. It's about keeping your energy levels up and staying healthy. Go for a walk with the stroller, do some home workouts, or join a dad's fitness group. Staying active will boost your mood, help you sleep better, and keep you in shape for all those future piggyback rides.

- **Eat Well.** Amidst the chaos, don't neglect your diet. Proper nutrition is needed to maintain your energy levels. Aim for balanced meals with lots of fruits, vegetables, lean proteins, and whole grains. And, of course, drink lots of water. Keep healthy snacks around so you're not tempted by those leftover baby biscuits. You can't run on coffee and baby food alone!

- **Your Mental Health.** It's normal to feel overwhelmed, anxious, or even a bit down at times. Make sure you take breaks and talk to someone about how you're feeling, be it your partner, family, a friend or a therapist. Find what helps you recharge, whether it's going for a run, chatting with your partner, or just a quiet moment to yourself. If things get too heavy, reach out for professional help. Your physical health is important, but so is your mental health. So, look after it! A happy, healthy dad makes for a happy, healthy family.

Dadhood is a marathon, not a sprint. Your health and well-being are just as important as your baby's. Taking care of yourself is vital for you to become the great dad you want to be!

Caring for baby, checking each sign,
You've got the rhythm; you're doing just fine.
Watching for giggles, feeling those kicks,
Vital signs checked, ever-ready with a fix.

Your emotional health is key, so get some rest too
Balancing stress and joy will do a world of good.
A little self-care and some breathing space,
Will help you keep up with the parenting race.

With love in your heart and patience to spare,
You're a rock for your little one, always there.
Baby's health, your wellness, a delicate dance,
But together, they'll thrive, if given a chance.

~ akin.o ~

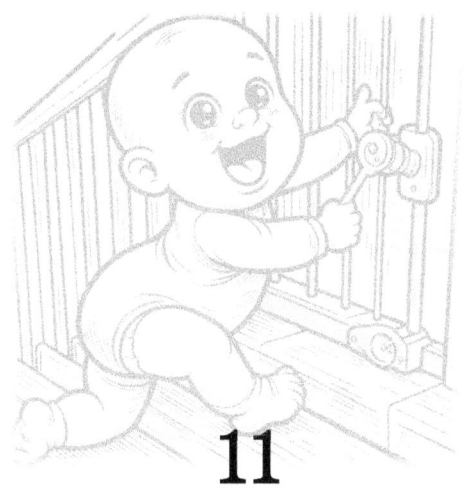

11

Safe and Secure
The Dadhood Edition

Mastering your baby's safety might sound like a tall order, but it's all about taking small, steady steps. From baby-proofing your home to baby-safe travel, you'll find that keeping your little one safe soon becomes second nature. Think of it as becoming a safety ninja - quick, vigilant, and always prepared to save the day!

Creating a Safe Haven

Your house might feel like a fortress, but to a curious baby, it's more of an amusement park full of potential hazards. So, before your little one starts crawling and exploring every nook and cranny, baby-proof your home. This might sound overkill, but you'll thank yourself later when your tiny tot cannot stick a fork in the socket or use the coffee table as a jungle gym. Here's a quick guide to making your home baby-safe without turning it into a sterile, boring, un-fun zone.

- **Cover Those Electrical Outlets.** Those tiny fingers have a knack for finding their way into electrical outlets. Invest in outlet covers or plates to keep your little explorer safe. It's a small investment for a big peace of mind. Remember, curiosity and electricity can be a dangerous combo!

- **Secure the Furniture.** That bookshelf might look solid, but to your baby, it's an open invitation to climb. Secure heavy furniture to the walls with brackets or straps. A toppled dresser is a disaster waiting to happen. Think of it as earthquake-proofing, minus the tectonic plates.

- **Mind the Corners and Edges.** Babies are like magnets to sharp edges. Coffee tables, fireplace hearths, and even those stylish chairs you love can become hazardous. Corner guards and edge bumpers can turn those potential noggin-busters into cushioned safety zones.

- **Keep Small Objects Out of Reach.** Babies love to put everything in their mouths. Coins, buttons, and basically anything smaller than a tennis ball are choking hazards. Keep these items out of reach, and do a daily scan of the floor for rogue objects that might have fallen.

- **The Hidden Dangers.** Kitchen knives, scissors, and even everyday objects like pens and pencils can become hazards. Store them out of reach or in locked drawers. For added safety, use blunt-tip scissors and safety knives when possible. Your baby will eventually grow curious about the kitchen, and it's best to be prepared.

- **Chemical Lockdown.** Cleaning supplies, medicines, and other hazardous materials should be stored out of reach or in locked cabinets. Install child-proof locks on cabinets and drawers. It's an extra step that may slow you down, but keep those little hands out of trouble. And don't forget about the garage, where chemicals like antifreeze or paint can be particularly dangerous.

- **Fire Safety.** This starts with prevention. Carry out monthly smoke detector checks and yearly battery changes - nothing ruins a nap like that relentless chirping. Keep fire extinguishers in key areas, like the kitchen and near the fireplace, and know how to use them. It may sound silly, but you may also want to practice fire drills. Trust me, your quick exit strategy is worth it.

- **Install Stair Gates.** Stairs are like Mount Everest to a baby: dangerous yet appealing. Stair gates at the top and bottom of your staircase can help prevent daring ascents or unintended descents. Make sure the gates are securely installed and always closed.

- **Cord Control.** Loose cords from blinds, curtains, or electronics are potential hazards. Keep them out of reach, or use cord winders to shorten them. Tuck away power strips and bundle cords together. Your baby's mission is to find them, and your job is to outsmart their tiny hands.

- **Water Safety.** This is not just for pools. An inch of water is enough for a baby to drown in, so be vigilant. Never leave a bucket of water or a filled bathtub unattended. Install child-proof toilet locks and keep bathroom doors closed. A curious baby can turn a seemingly harmless situation into a dangerous one in a flash.

- **Window Safety.** Keep windows secure and use window guards to prevent falls.

- **Pet Safety.** If you have pets, supervise their interactions with your baby. Even the friendliest pets can be unpredictable.

- **Routine Safety Checks.** Set monthly reminders to walk

through your home with a checklist, assessing any new risks or areas that might need adjustment. As your tiny explorer becomes more mobile, certain safety measures may need updating, fixing or even replacing. These small, consistent efforts ensure that your home remains a sanctuary for your baby as they grow and discover the world around them.

Baby-proofing isn't about wrapping your home in bubble wrap; it's about creating a safe environment where your baby can explore and grow. Remember, home safety is not a one-time task. Stay vigilant and adapt as your baby grows. So grab your tools, get down on all fours for a baby's-eye view, and turn your home into a safe haven where your little one can explore and thrive. Keep it safe, keep it secure, keep it fun, and try to stay one step ahead.

Sweet Dreams, Safe Slumbers

Sleep safety isn't just about getting some much-needed shut-eye yourself (though that's a huge bonus). It's about creating a safe environment for your baby to snooze in. Safe sleep is paramount for your baby's health, and here are a few ways to ensure that their sleeping environment is both comfortable and safe.

- **The Right Cot (Crib) Setup.** This might seem straightforward, but setting it up correctly is crucial for your baby's safety. Make sure the mattress is firm and fits snugly without gaps around the edges, and remove any pillows, toys, and blankets. Think of it as a minimalistic sleep sanctuary - anything else is just a party crasher.

- **Safe Sleep Positions.** Back is best! Always place your baby on their back to minimise the chance of Sudden Infant Death Syndrome (SIDS). While tummy time is excellent for playtime to build those muscles, bedtime is strictly a back affair. And no, your baby won't develop a flat head - that's just a myth.

- **Managing the Sleep Environment.** Keep the sleep environment cool and comfortable, around 20-22°C (68-72°F). Dress your baby in breathable, lightweight clothing to avoid overheating. A good rule of thumb is to dress them in one more layer than you'd wear yourself. No need to turn their room into a sauna - think cosy, not roasting.

- **Room Sharing, Not Bed Sharing.** For the first six months, keeping your baby's cot in your room is recommended. This reduces the risk of SIDS and makes nighttime feeds easier. Avoid bed-sharing - your bed is not designed to be baby-safe and can pose risks.

- **Gadgets and Gizmos.** There are tons of baby sleep gadgets out there, from white noise machines to sleep monitors. While they can be helpful, they're not substitutes for safe sleep practices. Use them as accessories, not crutches. And always read the instructions - no one wants a midnight gadget malfunction.

Remember, sleep safety is more than just avoiding hazards; it's about creating a peaceful environment where everyone can rest easy. So, set up that cot, check the temperature, and settle in for some well-deserved sleep. Sweet dreams!

Avoiding Food Fiascos

Feeding a baby has the tendency to be messy, but beyond the mess, there are safety concerns you need to be aware of. We're talking choking hazards, temperature checks, and how to handle your mini food critic. So, here are a few need-to-knows.

- **Introduction of Solids.** Once your baby hits the six-month mark, it's time to introduce solids. Think of it as the beginning of their culinary journey. Start with simple, single-ingredient purees like mashed bananas or sweet potatoes. Remember, you're not competing for a Michelin star here - simplicity is key. One day, you'll be a puree pro, but for now, revel in the chaos and mess.

- **Identifying Choking Hazards.** Babies have a knack for turning any meal into a potential hazard. Avoid foods like grapes, nuts, and popcorn - basically, anything that requires a full set of molars to chew. Cut food into little, manageable pieces, and always supervise your baby while they're eating. Choking hazards are real, but with a watchful eye, you can prevent any scares.

- **Safe Feeding Positions.** Finding the perfect feeding position can sometimes feel like an Olympic sport. Your baby should be seated upright, ideally in a highchair, to minimise the risk of choking and maximise comfort. And let's be honest, it's easier to clean up when they're in one spot rather than chasing them around the house with a spoon.

- **Temperature Checks.** Hot food is a big no-no. Always check the temperature of the food first before serving it to your baby. A quick taste test or using the back of your wrist will do the trick. Just make sure you're not caught stealing a bite of their apple puree - your little one can be surprisingly territorial.

- **Dealing with Your Mini Food Critic.** Babies are notorious for their fickle tastes. One day, they love carrots; the next day, they act like you've served them the worst meal ever. Keep offering a variety of foods, stay patient, and try not to take it personally. Remember, it's all part of their grand tasting adventure.

Feeding your baby is a journey filled with messes, milestones, and mini-victories. Embrace the process, keep it safe, and enjoy the delight of meal times.

Splash and Secure

Bathtime is one of the best bonding times, but it can sometimes be a tricky one. From water temperature to having everything you need within reach, here are a few ways to make sure bathtime is fun and safe.

- **Ideal Bath Temperature.** First things first: the water temperature. Aim for warm, not hot. The ideal bath temperature for your little one is about 37.8°C (100°F). Test it with your elbow or wrist - the water should feel comfortably warm, not scalding.

- **Never Leave the Baby Unattended.** This one's non-negotiable. Your baby can drown in as little as an inch of water. So, once your baby is in the tub, stay within arm's reach at all times. That text message can wait, and the phone call can go to voicemail. Your eyes are the best lifeguards.

- **Bath Time Essentials.** Ensure you have everything you need within arm's reach before you start the bath. This includes a soft towel, gentle baby soap, a clean diaper, and fresh clothes. The last thing you want is to start scrambling for a towel while your baby is doing their best impression of a slippery fish.

- **Get a Grip.** Babies are squirmy little creatures, especially when they're wet. A baby bath seat or non-slip mat can help keep things steady. It's like adding a bit of traction to your bathtime pit stop. And remember, a firm grip is key - you're handling precious cargo here.

- **Keep It Short and Sweet.** Babies have a short attention span, and their skin is sensitive. Aim for a bath time of about 5-10 minutes. This is plenty of time to get your baby clean without drying out their skin or turning bath time into a marathon.

- **Make It Fun.** Bathtime is a great bonding experience, so have fun with it. Sing songs, splash gently, and play with bath toys. Your baby will associate bathtime with positive memories, and you'll enjoy the bonding moment, too.

Bathtime should be a joy for both you and your baby, a time for fun and giggles. Hopefully, with these tips, you can safely grab that rubber ducky and enjoy the bathtime adventure.

Baby-Safe Travels

Whether it's a trip to the park or a long-haul flight, travelling with your mini-adventurer requires a new level of planning, preparation and precaution. Here's your mini guide to keeping things smooth and safe when you're on the move.

- **Car Seat Safety.** The key is to ensure the seat fits snugly in your car and is compatible with your vehicle's LATCH (Lower Anchors and Tethers for Children) system. This is your best friend when it comes to keeping the seat steady without using seat belts. You'll find anchors between the seat cushions in most cars, making installation easier and safer. Always follow the manufacturer's instructions meticulously. Regularly check that the car seat is secure and that the harness straps are correctly adjusted - they should sit at or below your baby's shoulders for rear-facing seats and at or above for forward-facing seats. Also, ensure that the chest clip rests at armpit level, not down by the belly. This positioning prevents the straps from slipping off in case of sudden stops. Use the "pinch test" to test the strap tightness. Pinch the strap at your baby's shoulder; if there's any excess webbing, then it's too loose. So, strap your baby in right, and cruise with peace of mind.

- **Never Alone.** This one is a no-brainer. Never leave your baby alone in the car. Even on mild days, cars can heat up quickly. So, always take your baby with you when you leave the vehicle.

- **Baby-Proof the Car.** Think of how your house is baby-proofed. Your car needs the same level of attention. Use cargo nets to store loose items securely to ensure they don't turn into dangerous projectiles in the event of a sudden stop. Window shades can keep the sun from turning your baby into a mini baked potato. And yes, snacks are essential - but choose non-choking hazards and have a plan for cleaning up the inevitable mess.

- **The Travel Essentials Checklist.** Packing for a trip with your little one is like preparing for a space mission. You'll need diapers, wipes, extra clothes, feeding supplies, and comfort items like their favourite toy or blanket. A portable changing pad is a lifesaver for those impromptu diaper changes in less-than-ideal locations. Keep a first-aid kit handy with baby-specific items, and don't forget to bring some entertainment for longer trips - think soft books, teething toys, and music.

- **Plan Breaks.** Long trips need careful scheduling. Plan breaks every two to three hours, allowing time for feeding, diaper changes, and stretching those tiny legs. It's all about keeping your baby comfortable and happy during the ride. Plus, a happy baby means a smoother drive for everyone involved.

- **Flying with Baby.** Taking to the skies? Where possible, book flights that align with your baby's sleep schedule. Invest in a baby carrier - it keeps your hands free and your baby close, which is especially useful during security checks. Offer a bottle or pacifier during takeoff and landing to help with ear pressure. And don't worry about the occasional cry - everyone's been there. A smile and an apology should sort that out.

- **Staying Calm and Flexible.** No matter how well you plan, travel with your baby is unpredictable. So, stay calm, be flexible, and remember that every hiccup is just part of the adventure. Laugh off the small stuff and focus on the memories you're making. After all, a baby with a passport is basically a future world explorer.

Travelling with your baby adds a layer of complexity, but it's also a fantastic opportunity for bonding and adventure. Remember, preparation is key. With the right preparation, you'll be able to travel like an expert in no time.

In a Nutshell

And there you have it – your simple guide to mastering your baby's health and safety. From bathtime to bedtime, feeding to first aid, and everything in between, you're now armed with the tips and tricks you need to ensure your little one grows up happy and healthy. Remember, it's all about the love, care, and attention you give every day. So, trust yourself, stay calm, and enjoy every precious moment with your little one.

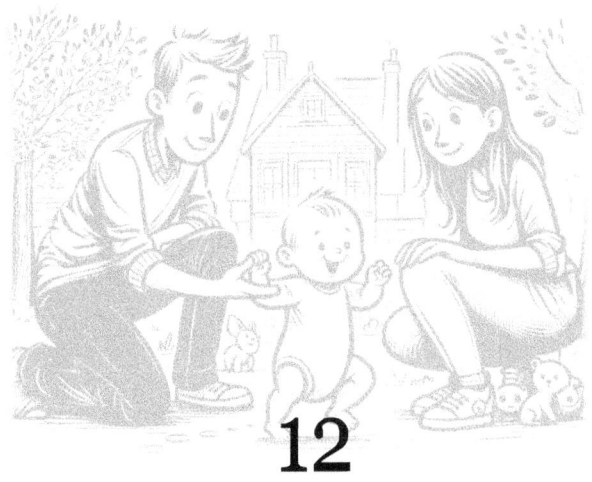

12

Baby's Greatest Hits
First-Year Milestones

Imagine yourself proudly watching your little munchkin as they navigate the realms of crawling, cruising, and eventually walking. It's like witnessing a miniature explorer charting new territories, and trust me, no matter how many maps you've got, each step is a brand-new adventure. These milestones are the greatest hits of babyhood, each one a testament to their incredible growth and budding independence. From tummy time to those wobbly first steps, I hope this chapter will help guide you through the first-year journey of your baby's physical development, ensuring you're ready to support and celebrate every precious moment.

Zero to Three Months: Survival Mode

The newborn stage, also known as the "Survival Mode" phase, is a whirlwind of sleepless nights, countless diaper changes, and trying to decode baby cues. But you can still expect so many cherishable moments like these:

- **Recognising Faces and Voices.** From the get-go, your baby starts recognising familiar faces and voices. They've spent months listening to your voice from the womb, so don't be surprised if they seem to respond to you from day one. Talk, sing, and make eye contact. Like we said before, these simple actions will help strengthen your bond and stimulate their developing brain.

- **First Social Smile.** Around six to eight weeks, or even earlier, you might witness the magical moment of your baby's first social smile. It's enough to melt your heart and make all those sleepless nights worth it. This smile is a sign that your baby is starting to engage with the world around them. So, get ready to whip out your camera and capture that gummy grin.

- **Object Grasping.** Your baby will begin to develop their motor skills, starting with grasping objects. At first, it's more of a reflex, but soon, they'll start to hold onto your finger or a rattle. It's a small step but a huge leap in their development. Encourage this by offering safe, baby-friendly objects for them to hold and explore.

Though this stage might seem chaotic, it's filled with unforgettable memories. So, Don't stress about creating a perfect routine. Simply embrace the moment, and try and get some rest when you can.

Three to Six Months: The Wiggle Phase

Now, here is where your baby starts gaining more control over their body and performing some serious moves. During this phase, they'll begin rolling over and even sitting up with some support, so be prepared to encourage their development. Also, get ready to take loads of pictures and a video recording or two because you can expect lots of this:

- **Rolling Over.** One of the first significant milestones in this phase is rolling over. It's your baby's first taste of mobility and independence. First, your baby will start to rock from side to side, and before you know it, they'll surprise you with a full roll. Make sure to capture that moment – it's pure gold. Create a safe space for tummy time to strengthen their neck and back muscles. And remember, once they start rolling, those ninja diaper changes get a little bit trickier.

- **Sitting with Support.** Your baby might start sitting up with some help. Propping them up with pillows or using a supportive baby seat can give them a new perspective on the world. Sitting up helps improve their balance and core strength, preparing them for crawling and beyond. It also frees up their hands to inevitably reach for your face. So, be ready for some joyful slapping!

- **Reach and Grab.** During this phase, your baby's hand-eye coordination takes a giant leap. They'll reach for toys, grab them, and maybe even pass them from one hand to the other. Try introducing colourful, textured toys that are safe for mouthing - because everything goes into their mouth. It's all part of their learning process.

Take in the excitement and discovery of this phase. Encourage your baby's movements and cheer them on. It's a time of rapid development and exploration. And remember, every wiggle, roll, and sit-up is a step towards their next big milestone.

Four to Six Months: The Soundtrack of Laughter

Get ready for one of the most joyous phases of your baby's first year - babbling and laughing! During this period, your baby's personality really starts to shine through their sounds and interactions. Here are a few things that make this phase so delightful:

- **Babbling and Cooing.** Your baby will start experimenting with sounds. Babbling and cooing become their favourite activities. You'll hear a symphony of "ba-ba-ba" and "ga-ga-ga" as they test out their vocal cords. It's their way of practising language, even if it sounds like they're speaking in tongues. Engage with them by mimicking their sounds and having "conversations." It helps them learn the basics of communication, and of course, it's a fun bonding activity.

- **First Laugh.** Nothing is more heartwarming than hearing your baby's first laugh. It might happen while you're playing peekaboo, making funny faces, or simply tickling their tummy. Baby laughter is contagious; making them giggle will likely become a daily goal. Apart from being adorable, it's also a sign that they're developing social and emotional skills.

- **Responding to Their Name.** Your baby starts to recognise their name and may respond to it. It's another huge milestone in their cognitive development. Try calling their name from different rooms and watch how they turn their head towards the sound. It's a clear sign they're recognising their identity and connecting it with you.

This phase is all about sound and interaction. Read to your baby, sing songs, and talk to them as much as possible. The more they hear, the more they'll want to mimic and join in. It's a noisy, laughter-filled time that lays the foundation for their future communication skills. Just make sure you have your camera at the ready, precious moments await.

Six to Nine Months: The Mobile Era

It's time for your baby to start crawling and turning into a tiny explorer – if they haven't already. During this stage, your little one's curiosity will know no bounds. Here are some tips to help support their newfound mobility:

- **Crawling and Scooting.** During this phase, your little one will likely start crawling, scooting, rolling, or even doing a combination of movements. Every baby has a unique style, and it's all about finding their way to get from point A to B. Encourage crawling by creating a safe space for them to practice their moves and placing toys just out of reach. Get ready to baby-proof everything, as their newfound mobility means they'll get into all sorts of adventures.

- **Pulling Up to Stand.** As their strength and confidence grow, your baby will start pulling up to stand. This might happen using furniture, your legs, or anything sturdy they can grab onto. It's a big step towards walking, and it's fascinating to watch them figure out how to balance. Make sure your furniture is secure, and consider installing corner protectors on sharp edges. Standing tall means many tumbles, so be ready to offer comforting hugs.

- **Furniture Cruising.** Once your baby masters pulling up, they'll begin cruising along furniture. This involves holding onto couches, tables, or anything within reach as they shuffle sideways. It's like their personal practice walking rail. Cheer them on and make sure the path is clear of obstacles. It won't be long before they let go and take those first independent steps.

This era is a thrilling time of growth and exploration. Let your baby explore safely and encourage their curiosity. Engage with them during playtime and watch as they learn and grow. Every crawl, stand, and cruise is a step towards greater independence and adventure. Cherish every moment, and I hope you still have that camera handy!

Six to Twelve Months: The Culinary Adventures

Welcome to the world of baby culinary adventures! This is when your baby's menu expands beyond milk, turning mealtime into a delightful and messy exploration. Introducing solids is massive, so here are a few tips to keep you on the right track:

- **Start with Purees.** Around six months, some earlier, your baby is ready to embark on their gastronomic journey. Begin with single-ingredient purees like mashed bananas, sweet potatoes, or avocado. These are easy on their tiny tummies and give them a taste of different flavours. Use a spoon to feed them, and watch as they hilariously scrunch up their faces while tasting new foods.

- **Explore Different Textures.** As your baby gets comfortable with purees, it's time to introduce a variety of textures. Gradually move from smooth purees to mashed and then finely chopped foods. This progression helps develop their chewing skills. Try offering small, soft pieces of fruit, cooked vegetables, and even tiny bits of well-cooked pasta. And yes, be prepared for the occasional food fight - it's all part of the fun.

- **Encourage Self-Feeding.** Around eight to nine months, your baby might show interest in self-feeding. Encourage this by offering finger foods like small pieces of soft fruit, cooked veggies, or cereal puffs. It's a messy endeavour but essential for developing their motor skills. Plus, watching them try to navigate food from plate to mouth with those chubby little hands is hilarious. Keep a bib and wipes handy!

- **Introducing Allergens.** Introduce common allergens like peanuts, eggs and dairy one at a time and observe for any reactions. Always consult your paediatrician for guidance. Introducing allergens at this early stage can help reduce the risk of developing food allergies.

The culinary adventure is an exciting time for you and your

baby. Enjoy the mess, celebrate the milestones, and savour the journey together, and as always, keep your camera handy for those priceless expressions. Bon appétit!

Nine to Twelve Months: Talking and Walking

This is a period filled with "Wow!" moments as your little one starts to find their voice and those adorable first words begin to emerge. You'll also witness those wobbly first steps that quickly turn into confident toddling.

First Words and Gestures

Get ready for a language explosion - your baby's about to become a tiny communicator! During this time, you'll witness the magic of first words and gestures as your little one starts to communicate more clearly. It's your job to try to understand and encourage their first words and gestures.

- **First Words.** Around nine to twelve months, your baby's babbling starts making sense. You'll likely hear those heart-melting first words like "Dada" or "Mama." – I don't know why, but for some reason "Dada" seems to come out first! Encourage their budding vocabulary by talking to them constantly, narrating your activities, and reading books together. Celebrate each new word with enthusiasm - it's a big deal!

- **Waving and Clapping.** Gestures are a significant part of early communication. Your baby might start waving hello and goodbye, imitating you and the social cues they observe. Clapping is another exciting milestone, often used to express joy or respond to your excitement. It's their way of joining in the fun and participating in social interactions. Keep the applause going - it's like their mini round of applause.

- **Pointing to Objects of Interest.** Your baby will begin pointing to objects they find interesting. It's like they're saying, "Hey, look at that!" or "I want that!" Responding to their pointing helps them feel understood and encourages more interaction. It's a great time to introduce new vocabulary - name the objects they're pointing to and watch their curiosity grow.

- **Encouraging Communication.** Create a language-rich environment by talking, singing, and playing with your baby. Use simple words, make eye contact, and give them time to respond. Interactive games like peekaboo or singing songs with actions can boost their communication skills. And remember, be patient - every baby develops at their own pace.

Like the other stages, the first words and gestures phase is an exciting time of discovery and interaction. Enjoy the chatter, celebrate the milestones, and keep those conversations flowing!

First Steps

Those first steps are simply monumental. You can expect your little one to go from standing to walking, turning your life into a delightful chase.

- **Standing Independently.** Once your baby can stand using furniture, your legs, or even the family dog for support, they'll start practising balancing and might even let go for a few wobbly seconds. It's an exciting time, and they'll be thrilled with their new perspective. Make sure you offer lots of encouragement and keep the camera ready - those wobbly stands are golden moments.

- **Taking First Steps.** The transition from standing to walking is a giant leap. Watching your baby take tentative steps between objects and then advancing to those magical first independent steps is priceless. Celebrate this milestone with lots of cheers and cuddles. Be prepared for some tumbles - bumps and bruises are part of the learning process. A soft play area can help cushion the sure-to-happen falls.

- **Transitioning from Crawling to Walking.** Walking is a whole new way for your baby to explore the world. They might switch back and forth between crawling and walking as they gain confidence. Encourage them to walk by holding their hands or using push toys. These help build strength and stability. And remember, once they're walking, nothing in your home is safe. So, baby-proofing becomes even more critical.

Watching your baby take their first steps is a proud and emotional experience. It's a reminder of how quickly they're growing and learning. Enjoy every moment, and don't worry about perfection - every stumble is a step towards mastering this new skill.

Capturing Special Moments

As your baby grows, every little achievement becomes a cherished memory. It's like watching a precious, tiny seed sprout and blossom into the most vibrant flower, each stage bringing new wonders. Celebrating your baby's first-year milestones is like celebrating small victories, each one worth remembering and cherishing. So, here's how we remember and celebrate these priceless moments:

- **Capture Every Moment You Can.** Make sure you capture everything you can. Whether it's their first wobbly step, smile, or giggle, keep your camera or smartphone handy. Snap candid shots, record videos, and don't worry about capturing the perfect moment - sometimes, the unplanned ones are the best. Photographs and videos instantly transport you back to those special days, so why not create a digital album or a physical scrapbook to organise these treasured memories. Just remember to back up those files - losing your baby's first giggle video is a nightmare no dad should face.

- **Keep a Milestone Journal.** Creating a milestone journal is priceless when it comes to documenting your baby's growth. Jot down each new skill or word, complete with dates and little anecdotes that capture the essence of the moment. Include little anecdotes or funny stories that accompany those milestones. This journal will become a treasured keepsake that you and your child can look back on together in the years to come. Plus, it's a great way to reflect on how much your baby has grown and changed.

- **Celebrate The Big and The Small.** Celebrate every milestone, big or small. Did your baby roll over for the first time, take their first step or say their first word? Break out the baby-safe cake and throw a mini party. Involving family and friends in these celebrations always adds another layer of joy. Recording and sharing these special moments with family and friends will create lasting memories for both you and your loved ones. By the way, these celebrations don't have to be elaborate or in-person. Sharing updates through family group chats or social media can keep everyone in the loop. A quick video clip or a few photos accompanied by a funny caption can spread smiles and excitement far and wide. It's about building a community of love and support around your little one and making these moments memorable.

- **Create Keepsakes and Traditions.** Consider creating keepsakes to commemorate significant milestones. Handprint and footprint kits, personalised baby blankets, or custom photo books are great options. These tangible items serve as beautiful reminders of your baby's early years and make excellent gifts for grandparents. Creating traditions around milestones can turn them into cherished family moments. Consider a first-year scrapbook, a family project that brings everyone together to curate the story of your baby's first year. Fill it with photos, notes, and little mementoes that capture the essence of each milestone. A growth chart wall in your home can be another delightful tradition. Each mark on the wall not only tracks your baby's physical growth but also serves as a visual journey of their development. These Keepsakes and traditions become part of your family's unique story, nurturing a sense of belonging and continuity.

- **Deep Reflections.** Reflecting on your baby's growth and development over the first year can be a deeply rewarding experience. Writing letters to your child about their growth can be a touching way to capture your thoughts and feelings. Share the joy you feel watching them grow, the challenges you've faced, and the hopes you hold for their future. These letters are a gift, a window into their early years that they can cherish as they grow older. And while reflecting on their growth, take a moment to consider your own journey as a dad. Discuss your personal growth with your partner, acknowledging how your baby has shaped and enriched your life. These reflections foster an appreciation for the incredible bond you've built and the adventure that lies ahead.

Your baby's first year is like a hit parade of heart-warming moments and tiny triumphs. From those first sleepy smiles to the day they start toddling around like they own the place, each milestone is a standing ovation in the concert of their life. It's a whirlwind of emotions, filled with laughter, surprises, and, most likely, a few sleepless nights. But through it all, you're building memories that will bring a smile to your face for years to come. Remember, these moments, both big and small, are the threads that weave together the tapestry of your family's story. So keep that camera ready and cherish every little "first" because these are the days you'll look back on and realise they were the greatest hits of all.

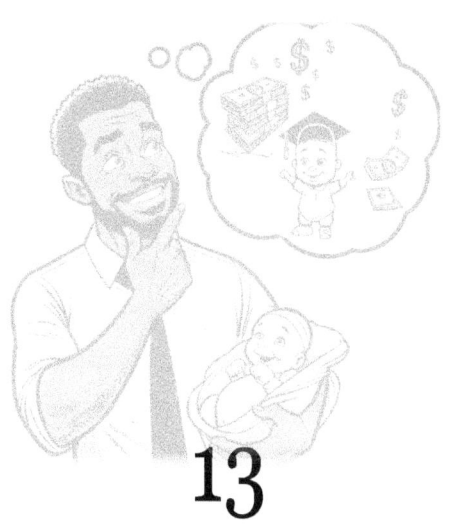

13

Growing Your Baby's Wealth
Savings, Investments and Education

So, with your little one on the way (or maybe already here), you'll find yourself thinking about things like savings accounts, college or university funds, investments, and so on. This might seem overwhelming at first, especially if you're juggling midnight feedings, diaper changes and other activities, but don't worry – I've got a few tips to help you along the way. Financial planning doesn't have to be overly complicated or stressful - I wish I had known this back then! With some organisation and smart choices, you can set your baby up for a secure and bright future.

Set Goals and Priorities

Kicking off the financial planning journey for your baby can feel like stepping into the unknown. But don't worry; it's more about setting relaxed, manageable goals and getting your priorities straight than diving into complex financial jargon. Think of it as mapping out a fun road trip where you decide the stops along the way.

- **Define Your Objectives.** This is the first step in your financial journey, like setting your GPS. Whether you're saving for your child's education, building an emergency fund, or both, pinpointing your aims helps create a clear, effective plan to guide your decisions and keep you on track.

- **Short-term vs. Long-term Goals.** Short-term and long-term goals are like two sides of the same coin, both essential but serving different purposes. Break down your goals into short-term (1-5 years) and long-term (5+ years) objectives. Short-term goals, like saving for childcare expenses or a family vacation, keep you motivated and give you quick wins. Long-term goals, on the other hand, are the big-ticket items like your child's education or buying a house. Balancing both helps ensure you're making progress now while keeping an eye on the future. It's all about finding that sweet spot between immediate needs and future dreams.

- **Estimate Costs.** This is like getting a sneak peek at the financial road ahead. Whether you're saving for your child's education, a new hobby, or even that dream family vacation, having a ballpark figure helps you plan better. It's about figuring out what you'll need and when so you're not caught off guard. Take a relaxed approach – you've already jotted down your goals, so do some research and see what each one will cost. This way, you can set realistic savings targets and make the journey to reaching them much smoother.

Build an Emergency Fund

This is like a financial safety net designed to catch you when life throws a curveball. It's all about making sure you're prepared for life's little surprises.

- **Why You Need an Emergency Fund.** Life is unpredictable. Having an emergency fund ensures you're prepared for any unexpected expenses, whether it's a sudden job loss, medical bills, or an urgent home repair; having a stash of cash set aside means you won't have to scramble or stress. It's about knowing that you're covered for life's little surprises.

- **How Much to Save.** Figuring out how much to save can feel like solving a puzzle, but it's simpler than you think. Aim to tuck away six months' worth of living expenses in your emergency fund. I know this sounds like a lot, but don't stress. Whether you save a little each week or set aside a lump sum when you can, every bit helps prepare you and your family for any financial hiccups.

- **Where to Keep It.** Choosing where to save your emergency fund is like finding the perfect spot for your nest egg to grow while staying safe. High-yield savings accounts are usually a top pick because they offer better interest rates than regular ones, meaning your money can grow faster. Plus, it's easy to access when needed without the risk of market fluctuations.

Start a Savings Account

Starting a savings account for your baby is one of the simplest yet most impactful steps you can take towards securing their financial future. Think of it as planting a money tree that will grow as they grow. Whether you go for a high-yield savings account or a more specialised option, you're setting the groundwork for a solid financial foundation.

Types of Savings Accounts

When saving for your baby's future, choosing the right type of savings account is like picking the best tool for the job.

Whether you're looking at a Junior ISA, a Children's Savings Account, or a Trust Fund if you're in the UK, or 529 plans, a custodial account or a high-yield savings account if you live across the pond, each has its own benefits that can be tailored to suit your needs. Let's take a relaxed stroll through the various options available.

- **Junior ISA (JISA).** This is a fantastic way to save for your child's future in a tax-free environment. It's like giving their savings a head start right from the get-go. You can choose between the Cash and Stocks & Shares options, whichever best meets your needs. The best part? Your child can't access the money until they turn 18, ensuring it grows undisturbed for years. So, whether you're saving for university fees or just a financial cushion, a JISA can be a great option to consider.

- **Children's Savings Account.** A Children's Savings Account is a great starter option for your little one's financial journey. It's straightforward, easy to set up, and helps get them into the habit of saving from an early age. While it might not offer the tax perks of a Junior ISA, it's still a fantastic way to watch those pennies grow. Plus, many banks offer fun incentives for kids, making the whole experience enjoyable for them. So, if you're looking for a good option for saving smaller amounts, a Children's Savings Account is a solid choice.

- **529 College Savings Plans.** This is a fantastic way to stash away funds for your child's future education. Think of it as a dedicated piggy bank that grows over time. These plans grow tax-free, and you won't pay taxes on withdrawals as long as they're used for qualified education expenses. You can even choose from a variety of investment options based on your risk tolerance.

- **UGMA (Uniform Gifts to Minors Act) and UTMA (Uniform Transfers to Minors Act).** Custodial Accounts are great ways to save and invest for your child's future. Think of them as a financial toolkit where you can stash money, stocks, bonds, and even real estate. The account grows in the child's name but is under your control until they hit the age of majority, usually 18 or 21. It's a flexible and easy way to manage assets for your kiddo's future.

- **High-Yield Savings Accounts.** These are like the overachievers of the banking world. They offer better interest rates than your typical savings accounts, helping your money grow faster without any extra effort. Whether you're saving for a rainy day or your baby's future, these accounts give you more bang for your buck. Plus, they're usually as easy to manage as regular savings accounts. So, if you want your money to work a little harder for you, high-yield savings accounts are definitely worth looking at.

Investing for Your Child's Future

This might sound like a big task, but think of it as planting a tree that'll grow alongside your child, providing shade and fruit in the years to come. It's all about setting aside a bit of money now to ensure they have a secure and prosperous future. Whether you're looking at stocks, bonds, mutual funds, or even something more conservative, there are plenty of ways to make your money work harder for your little one. Here are some smart and straightforward strategies to help you build that financial nest egg with confidence and ease.

- **Stocks and Shares ISA (UK).** Think of this as a tax-efficient way to dip your toes into the stock market. With this type of ISA, your money can grow through investments in stocks, bonds, and funds, all while enjoying tax-free returns. It's a bit like giving your child's savings a turbo boost. A Stocks and Shares ISA is a solid option if you want to build a robust financial cushion for your little one's future.

- **Bonds and Gilts (UK).** These are fixed-income investments. They are a solid, straightforward way to invest for your child's future. Whether government or corporate, bonds and gilts offer stable returns and are a great way to balance out riskier investments like stocks. Government gilts are said to be very safe, but they generally offer lower returns compared to stocks. Think of bonds and gilts as the reliable, steady growers in your investment garden, providing a dependable foundation for your child's financial future.

- **Unit Trusts (UK).** Investing in Unit Trusts is like teaming up with other investors to buy a diverse portfolio of assets managed by a professional. It's a great way to get a slice of the investment pie without having to pick individual stocks or bonds yourself. Unit Trusts spread the risk across various assets, which can provide a more stable return over time. So, whether you're new to investing or just looking for a straightforward option, Unit Trusts can be a solid choice to help grow your child's financial future.

- **Mutual Funds and Exchange-Traded Funds (ETFs).** These are like the trusty sidekicks of the investment world, perfect for building a diverse portfolio without the stress of picking individual stocks yourself. These funds pool your money with other investors, spreading it across various assets managed by professionals. This diversification helps balance risk and can provide more stable returns over time. Whether you're a newbie investor or just looking for an easy way to grow your child's savings, mutual funds and ETFs are solid, hassle-free options to help secure your little one's financial future.

- **Stocks and Bonds (USA).** Investing in stocks and bonds for your child's future is like creating a balanced diet for their financial health. Stocks can provide the high-growth potential needed to build wealth over time but come with higher risk, while bonds offer stability and lower but steady returns. Combining these two allows you to create a diversified portfolio that balances risk and reward. It's a straightforward strategy that can help ensure your child's savings grow steadily, giving you peace of mind as you watch their financial future flourish.

- **Index Funds (USA).** Index funds are like the steady workhorses of the investment world. They track a specific market index and provide an affordable way to invest in a broad range of stocks. This means you get diversification and reduced risk without having to pick individual stocks. Over the long term, index funds tend to perform well, making them a solid choice for growing your child's savings. So, if you're looking for a straightforward, hassle-free investment option, index funds might be the way to go.

Education Savings Plans

When it comes to securing your child's future, education savings plans are like giving them a head start in the financial marathon. These plans are designed to help you save for those big educational expenses down the road, often with some sweet tax benefits thrown in. The key is to start early and let the magic of compound interest do its thing. So, let's explore how these plans can turn your savings into a bright educational future for your little one.

- **Junior ISA (JISA).** As mentioned earlier, this is a great way to save for your child's education without the tax worries. It's like giving your child's savings a little extra boost, as any interest or investment gains within a JISA grow tax-free. You can choose between a Cash JISA, which offers steady returns, or a Stocks and Shares JISA, which has the potential for higher growth. You can contribute up to £9,000 per year (as of 2025) without paying any tax on the interest or investment gains. The money is locked in until your child turns 18, so it has plenty of time to grow and provide the perfect financial foundation for those future education costs.

- **Regular Savings Plans.** These are like the steady drumbeat of your financial planning for your child's education. With these plans, you consistently set aside a bit of money each month - this could be a monthly direct debit into a savings or investment account - making it easier to build up a significant fund over time. Whether you choose a high-interest savings account or a dedicated education savings plan, the key is consistency. Over the years, those regular contributions can really add up, giving you peace of mind and ensuring your little one has the funds they need for their educational journey.

- **529 College Savings Plans.** Also mentioned earlier, a 529 plan is an excellent way to save for your child's education with tax benefits. These plans are like dedicated piggy banks that grow over time, offering tax-free growth on your contributions and withdrawals for qualified education expenses. With various investment options tailored to your risk tolerance, a 529 plan makes saving for future tuition bills easy and efficient. There are two types of 529 plans:

    - **Prepaid Tuition Plans.** These allow you to lock in today's prices for tomorrow's education - a real win-win for your wallet. With these plans, you can purchase future tuition credits at current rates, protecting you from the rising cost of college tuition. It's like securing an early bird special for your child's education. These plans are perfect if you have a good idea of where your child might attend college.

    - **Education Savings Plans.** These are like the ultimate toolbox for funding your child's education, offering both prepaid tuition plans and education savings plans. It allows you to invest your money in various options, ranging from conservative to aggressive, based on your risk appetite. These plans grow tax-free, and you won't pay taxes on withdrawals as long as they're used for qualified education expenses. It's a flexible and efficient way to build a solid financial foundation for your child's academic future.

- **Coverdell Education Savings Accounts (ESA).** This is like a trusty sidekick for your child's educational journey. With this account, you can save up to $2,000 per year per child, and the funds grow tax-free. While it has lower contribution limits than a 529 plan, it offers more flexibility in terms of how the funds can be used, including for K-12 expenses. Whether it's for tuition, books, or even some tech gadgets, a Coverdell ESA is a flexible and tax-friendly way to ensure your child has the financial support they need for their learning adventures.

So, the game plan to secure your baby's financial future is in motion. By setting goals and priorities, building that trusty emergency fund, opening a savings account, and investing wisely, you're setting your little one on the path to success. But we're not done yet.

You're on a mission, planning with care,
Building baby's wealth, always aware.
Emergency funds for rainy days,
Saving and investing, in many wise ways.

Stocks and bonds, and piggy banks full,
To help little one prosper in all they do.
Education funds and life skills, too,
With every penny saved, dreams come true.

Teaching lessons, money smarts,
Dad's guidance is where it starts.
With love and foresight, baby's wealth will grow,
And by His grace, baby's life will glow!

~ akin.o ~

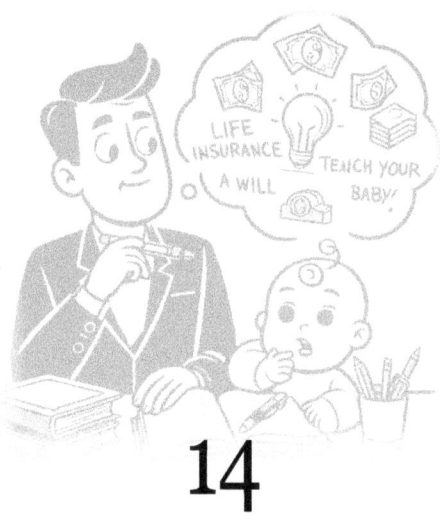

14

Future-Proofing Your Little One
Tax Tips, Life Insurance, and More

As we continue on the journey to securing your baby's financial future, let's look at a few more steps you can take to help with their financial stability and also offer peace of mind. We're talking about maximising available tax benefits, securing life insurance, and even creating a will. Oh, and let's not forget the importance of teaching your little one how to be money-savvy.

Maximising Tax Benefits

Maximising tax benefits can sometimes feel like finding hidden treasures. There are quite a few ways to keep more of your hard-earned money while securing your child's future. It's all about being savvy and taking advantage of all the child tax credits and deductions available to you.

- **Child Benefit (UK).** This provides a regular payment to help with the costs of raising a child. It's available to most parents or guardians and can make a real difference in covering everyday expenses. You can claim Child Benefit for each child under your care. And since it isn't means-tested, there's a possibility that you'll be eligible. It's like getting a helping hand from the government to give your baby the best start in life.

- **Tax-Free Childcare (UK).** If you and your partner both work, you may be eligible for Tax-Free Childcare. This government scheme helps working parents by providing up to £2,000 per year per child to cover childcare costs. It's pretty straightforward - for every £8 you pay into your childcare account, the government adds an extra £2. These funds can be used for various childcare providers, from nurseries to after-school clubs. Taking advantage of this benefit can ease the financial burden of childcare, making it easier to balance work and family life.

- **Earned Income Tax Credit (EITC).** This is like a little financial gift for working parents in the USA. It's a refundable tax credit designed to help low to moderate-income families by reducing the amount of tax owed and potentially giving you a nice refund. If you qualify, it can provide a significant boost to your household budget, easing financial strain and giving you more resources to support your baby. So, check your eligibility and take advantage of this helpful tax benefit to maximise your financial planning efforts.

- **Dependent Care Tax Credit.** The Dependent Care Tax Credit is another little financial lifesaver for working parents in the USA. This credit can help offset the cost of childcare expenses if you're working or looking for work. By claiming this credit, you can get a percentage of your childcare expenses back as a tax refund, which can significantly lighten the financial load. It's a great way to ease the burden of childcare costs and ensure you're making the most of the tax benefits available to you.

Life Insurance

When it comes to securing your baby's future, life insurance might not be the first thing that pops into your mind, but it's a cornerstone of a solid financial plan. Think of it as a security blanket, providing financial protection for your family in case of unforeseen events.

- **Why Life Insurance Matters.** Life insurance ensures that your loved ones are taken care of, covering expenses like daily living costs, education, and even future dreams. It's all about knowing that your family's financial future is safeguarded no matter what life throws your way.

- **Types of Life Insurance.** There are various life insurance options, each offering unique benefits to suit different needs. Understanding the multiple options available can help you make the best choice. In the UK, we've got:

    - **Term Life Insurance.** Covers you for a set period (like 20 or 30 years). Ideal for covering things like your mortgage.

    - **Whole Life Insurance.** This offers lifelong coverage with a savings component that grows over time.

    - **Critical Illness Insurance.** Pays out if you're diagnosed with a serious illness. It helps to cover medical expenses.

    - **Income Protection Insurance.** Provides regular income if you're unable to work because of illness or injury.

    - **Over 50s Life Insurance.** Available to those aged 50 and over. No medical exam is required.

- **Joint Life Insurance.** Covers two people and pays out on the first death. It's perfect for couples.

In the USA, we have:

- **Term Life Insurance.** This provides protection for a defined term (like 10, 20, or 30 years) and is generally more affordable.

- **Whole Life Insurance.** This option offers financial protection for your entire life with a savings component that grows over time.

- **Universal Life Insurance.** Similar to whole life but with flexible premiums and adjustable death benefits.

- **Variable Life Insurance.** This option combines life insurance with investment options, allowing the cash value to grow based on market performance.

- **Simplified Issue Life Insurance.** Quick approval without a medical exam, but typically more expensive.

- **Guaranteed Issue Life Insurance.** There's no need for a medical exam or health questions with this option. It's ideal for those with health issues but has higher premiums.

- **Choosing the Right Policy.** Start by considering your family's needs and financial goals. Are you looking for short-term coverage or something that will last a lifetime? Do you want a policy that includes investment components or something simpler like term life insurance? Think about the flexibility, cost, and benefits of each option. By matching the policy to your needs, you can ensure you're making a smart, well-informed decision. Having coverage 10-12 times your annual income is often recommended.

Creating a Will

This might not be the most exciting part when it comes to financial planning for your baby, but it's incredibly important. Once again, it's all about making sure your loved ones are cared for, no matter what the future holds. So, let's get into the nitty-gritty of securing your family's financial future.

- **Why You Need a Will.** A will guarantees that your assets are allocated according to your preferences and, if needed, that your child is looked after by a guardian of your choice. Without a will, the state determines how your assets are divided, which may not reflect your desires.

- **Choosing a Guardian.** Guardian selection for your child is akin to choosing a superhero who will step in if you or your partner are not around. It's a deeply personal decision that ensures your little one is cared for by someone you trust and who shares your values. Think about family members or close friends who have a strong bond with your child and can provide a loving, stable environment. Discuss your choice with them to ensure they're up for the responsibility. This way, you know your child will be in good hands, no matter what.

- **Setting Up Trusts.** Trusts are valuable tools for managing and safeguarding your assets for your child's future. They enable you to allocate assets and funds for your child's benefit. They are overseen by a trustee until a specific age or milestone is reached. They can also provide specific instructions on how and when the funds should be used. It's a flexible and efficient way to provide for your child's education, living expenses, or any special needs they may have.

Teaching Financial Literacy

Ensuring your child is financially literate is like giving them a superpower that will last a lifetime. It's about making money concepts fun and easy to understand and helping your child develop healthy financial habits.

- **Start Early.** Teaching financial literacy from a young age is akin to planting a seed that will flourish into a robust money tree. Introducing basic money concepts to your child at an early stage helps them cultivate smart money habits from the get-go. Use simple, fun lessons and everyday activities like grocery shopping or saving pocket money to teach them about budgeting, saving, and the value of money.

- **Use Tools and Resources.** Using tools and resources to teach financial literacy can make learning about money fun and engaging for your child. From colourful piggy banks and savings charts to interactive apps and games, there are plenty of ways to bring budgeting, saving, wise spending and other financial concepts to life. You can even use storybooks that teach money lessons in a playful way. By incorporating these tools into everyday life, you'll help your child understand the value of money, which will serve them well in the future.

- **Lead by Example.** This is one of the most powerful ways to teach financial literacy to your child. Children learn a lot by observing. When you handle money responsibly, discuss your budgeting decisions openly, and show the importance of saving, your child absorbs these habits naturally. Whether sticking to a grocery budget, saving for a family holiday, or making thoughtful spending choices, your actions speak louder than words.

Final Nuggets

Financial planning for your baby's future is an ongoing journey that requires careful thought and consistent effort. You can provide your child with a secure and promising future by setting clear goals, building a strong foundation with savings and investments, and using tax benefits and educational plans. I know it's a lot to take in but hang in there. Remember, start early and stay committed. Your efforts today will pay off in the long run, ensuring your little one has the opportunities they need to thrive.

Planning for the future, you're on the case,
Building a foundation, setting the pace.
With a wink and a smile, you chart the way,
Future-proofing your baby, come what may.

Teaching wisdom, sharing the lore,
You've got the roadmap; you're ready to explore.
With love and foresight, in every single deed,
You're future-proofing your baby, planting the seed!

~ akin.o ~

15

Mastering the Juggle
Work and Dadhood

So, there you are, working from home, trying to concentrate on the tasks before you, while your toddler is determined to share their newfound ability to sing the alphabet backwards. Welcome to the world of work and dadhood, where multitasking reaches new heights, and every day feels like a reality show episode you never signed up for. But I thought they said dads can't multitask. Well, I know we can! Mastering this juggle is entirely within your grasp, even if you sometimes feel like a circus performer without the safety net. Balancing work and family life is like walking a tightrope, but with these practical tips, I'm sure you'll find that sweet spot.

Set Priorities

Understanding and setting your priorities as a first-time dad can feel like juggling flaming torches while riding a unicycle. How do you figure out what matters most, and how do you allocate your time accordingly?

- **Identify Non-Negotiables.** First things first, figure out your non-negotiables. These are the things that matter most and aren't up for debate. Maybe it's being home for bedtime stories every night or making sure you hit the gym several times a week. Whatever they are, identify them and make sure they're non-negotiable. Write them down if you have to - it's a great way to remind yourself of what truly matters.

- **Balance Work Demands with Family Needs.** It's all about finding a balance that doesn't leave you feeling like you're shortchanging one or the other. Set workplace boundaries - communicate with your employer about your new responsibilities at home. Maybe that means not checking emails or arranging flexible working hours after a certain time. The goal is to be fully present wherever you are, whether it's at your work desk or on the living room floor building a LEGO castle.

- **Create a Priority List.** At the beginning of each week, jot down what's important. Rank them in order of importance and tackle them one by one. This helps ensure you're focusing on what really matters and not just putting out fires. And don't forget to include some 'me time' in there - after all, a well-rested dad is a happy dad.

- **Adjust as You Go.** Life is unpredictable, especially with a baby. Your priorities might need to shift on the fly, and that's okay. Be flexible and adjust as needed. The key is to stay focused on what's important and not get bogged down by the little stuff. Remember, it's all about progress, not perfection.

When you set priorities, you stay focused on what really matters. Identify your non-negotiables, balance work and family, create a priority list, and be ready to adjust. Keep juggling those flaming torches.

Become a Scheduling Ninja

Balancing work, baby, and some personal time requires serious scheduling skills. Well, say goodbye to chaos and hello to productivity. It's time to master the art of time management with strategies to make the most of your day.

- **Effective Planning and Scheduling.** A well-thought-out plan is your secret weapon. Start by setting a weekly schedule and noting all your essential tasks and appointments. A digital calendar or an old-fashioned manual planner - whatever works for you – should do the trick. The key is to have a clear view of what's coming up so nothing sneaks up on you. Maybe using a priority matrix could be the way to go. This visual tool is like having a GPS for your day. It keeps you on track even when life throws unexpected detours your way.

- **Time-Blocking Techniques.** Once you've sorted your tasks, you can allocate specific time blocks not just for work meetings and doctor's appointments, but family time, date nights, and some downtime for yourself. The idea is to compartmentalise your day so you're not constantly switching between tasks. It helps you stay focused and makes your day feel more manageable.

- **Find Time for Both Work and Play.** It's crucial to strike a balance between work and play. Too much of one can lead to burnout or feeling out of touch with family. Schedule your work hours and stick to them. Then, set aside time each day to spend with your family - whether it's playing with the baby, having dinner together, or just chatting about your day. Also, don't forget to carve out some personal time. A 30-minute break to read a book or take a walk can do wonders for your mental health.

- **Handling Distractions.** Distractions are inevitable, but managing them is crucial. If you're working from home, create a dedicated workspace and set boundaries with family members during work hours. Use productivity tools like noise-cancelling headphones, apps that block social media, and timers to keep you on track. And don't forget to take short breaks - just make sure you get back to work afterwards.

- **Embracing Flexibility.** Parenthood is unpredictable, and sometimes, your well-laid plans will go out the window. Embrace flexibility and be ready to adapt. If your baby's nap schedule changes or a work deadline shifts, adjust your plan accordingly. The ability to pivot is what makes a true time management ninja.

Mastering time management is all about effective planning, time-blocking, balancing work and play, handling distractions, and embracing flexibility. If you get this right, it's unlikely for work to seep into family time and you'll be fully present when you're with your loved ones.

Roll with the Punches

Dadhood is full of surprises, so flexibility and adaptability are your best friends when handling the unexpected.

- **Embrace a Fluid Schedule.** Your baby has their own schedule and is not particularly concerned with yours. Whether it's a sudden nap strike, an unplanned diaper blowout, or an unexpected meltdown in the grocery store, being able to adapt is key. Embrace the unpredictable and learn to go with the flow. A rigid schedule is a recipe for frustration. So, aim for a fluid routine that allows for adjustments. When things don't go as planned, take a deep breath and adjust your approach. The goal is to have a structure that bends and flexes with the day's whims.

- **Handle Last-Minute Work or Family Demands.** Work and family can throw you last-minute curveballs. Maybe your boss needs an urgent report, or your partner has a sudden craving for an obscure snack. Learn to prioritise and juggle these demands without losing your cool. It's okay to say "no" or ask for help when needed. Flexibility also means recognising your limits and knowing when to delegate.

- **Keep a Positive Attitude.** Flexibility isn't just about actions - it's also about mindset. Maintaining a positive attitude in the face of unexpected changes can make a huge difference. Instead of getting frustrated when plans go awry, try to see it as an adventure. Laugh off the little mishaps and focus on the big picture. Remember, it's the journey, not the destination.

Flexibility is all about dealing with each situation that is thrown your way and maintaining a positive attitude. Adjust to unexpected changes, embrace a fluid schedule, handle last-minute demands gracefully, and celebrate small wins.

Protect Your Personal Time

Establishing boundaries as a first-time dad might seem like a tall order, but it's crucial for maintaining your sanity and well-being. You need to carve out some personal time while trying your best to keep everyone happy.

- **Set Work Hours and Stick to Them.** One of the most critical aspects of protecting your personal time is setting clear work hours and sticking to them. When you're off the clock, be genuinely off the clock. This means shutting down your laptop, silencing work notifications, and resisting the urge to sneak a peek at emails. Let your colleagues know your availability and respect those boundaries yourself. It's like a digital "Do Not Disturb" sign.

- **Create a Dedicated Workspace.** Having a dedicated workspace when working from home can help maintain boundaries. This doesn't mean you need a fancy home office, just a designated work spot. When you leave that space, mentally clock out. It helps create a clear separation between work time and personal time. Plus, when you're in that space, it signals to your family that you're in work mode.

- **Communicate Your Boundaries.** For boundaries to be effective, they need to be communicated clearly. In a work situation, talk to your employer about your needs and negotiate flexible working arrangements when required. Similarly, discuss your boundaries with your partner and family. Explain why personal time is essential and how it benefits everyone. Encourage them to support you in maintaining these boundaries and offer to do the same for them.

- **Handle Boundary Pushers.** There will always be people or situations that push your boundaries. Stay firm but kind. If a colleague tries to rope you into after-hours work, politely remind them of your availability. If family demands encroach on your personal time, gently but firmly reinforce your need for that space. It's all about balance and respect.

- **Maintain Your Identity.** Becoming a dad doesn't mean abandoning who you are. Maintaining your identity and interests is essential to stay balanced and fulfilled. Don't neglect personal time and keep those social circles alive; they are key to balancing personal pursuits and dadhood. Remember, prioritising your well-being enriches not just your life but the lives of those you love.

Setting boundaries is essential for maintaining your personal time and well-being. Establish clear work hours, create a dedicated workspace, communicate with your employer and family, schedule personal time, and handle boundary pushers gracefully. Keep that balance in check.

Let Go of the Pressure

Dadhood often comes with a side dish of guilt for most dads - whether it's missing a milestone or feeling you're not doing enough. So, how do you handle the guilt and let go of the pressure?

- **Recognise It, Address It.** Every dad experiences guilt in some form, even those picture-perfect dads on social media. Recognising guilt is the first step to addressing it. Instead of letting it fester, confront it. Ask yourself why you're feeling guilty and whether it's justified. Often, guilt comes from unrealistic expectations - cut yourself some slack.

- **Be Realistic.** Overcoming guilt starts with adjusting your expectations. You're not a superhero. You're a human being doing your best. Set realistic goals and remember that it's okay to ask for help. Talking to someone can sometimes lighten the load. So share those feelings with your partner or a trusted friend. Practice self-compassion and remind yourself that nobody gets everything right all the time. Celebrate the things you're doing well instead of focusing on perceived shortcomings.

- **Quality Time Over Quantity.** It's easy to feel guilty about not spending enough time with your baby, especially if you're juggling work and other responsibilities. Focus on quality over quantity. A few minutes of undivided attention, playtime, or reading together can be more meaningful than hours of distracted presence. Make your time with your baby count, and let go of the guilt about the hours you can't be there.

- **Bye Bye Perfection.** A perfect dad doesn't exist. Social media can make it seem like everyone else has it all together, but remember that people often only share the highlights. Understand that mistakes are part of the journey and embrace the imperfections. Laugh off the mishaps and learn from them. Your baby needs love, care, and attention - not perfection.

- **Prioritise Self-Care.** Taking care of yourself isn't selfish; it's essential! Prioritising self-care helps you be a better parent. Whether taking a break, pursuing a hobby, or just having some quiet time, self-care recharges your batteries. When you're well-rested and happy, you'll be more present and effective as a dad.

Handling guilt is about recognising it, setting realistic expectations, focusing on quality time, letting go of perfection, and prioritising self-care. Embrace the journey, imperfections and all.

Reflect and Adjust

Work-life balance isn't a one-time achievement; it's an ongoing journey. Reflecting on your journey and making the necessary adjustments is the key to keeping things on track.

- **Regular Adjustments.** Dadhood isn't a set-it-and-forget-it deal. Regular check-ins with yourself and your partner help keep things balanced. Regularly take time to reflect on what's working and what's not. Are those late-night feedings running smoothly, or is your sleep schedule in shambles? Talk it out, make a plan, and adjust as needed. Think of it as a regular tune-up for your dadhood engine.

- **Set New Goals and Priorities.** As your baby grows, your priorities will shift. What was important last month might not be as crucial now. Set new goals and priorities to match your family's current needs. Maybe it's time to focus on sleep training, or perhaps it's about introducing solids. Keeping your goals flexible and adaptable means you'll always be moving forward. And don't forget to celebrate those little victories along the way.

- **Learn from Mistakes.** Mistakes are part of the journey. Maybe you forgot to pack an extra diaper, or bedtime turned into a marathon of tears. It happens. Instead of beating yourself up, learn from these moments. Reflect on what went wrong and how you can do better next time. Remember, dadhood doesn't come with a manual; it's all about trial and error.

- **Stay Flexible and Adaptable.** Kids grow, schedules change, and life throws curveballs. Being adaptable helps you navigate these changes with grace. Don't be afraid to pivot when needed. Embrace change and see each new challenge as an opportunity to learn and grow.

Reflecting and adjusting is an ongoing process that keeps you on top of your dadhood game. Regular check-ins, setting new goals, celebrating successes, learning from mistakes, and staying flexible are all part of this journey. Keep moving forward, and enjoy the ride.

Parental Leave: The Fears, the Joys and the Realities

I believe taking parental leave as a first-time dad is one of the best decisions you can make. It allows you to step away from work pressures and focus on family. It's a time to hit pause on the grind and dive headfirst into the beautiful chaos of dadhood. Imagine being there for all those firsts - first smile, first bath, first sleepless night (okay, maybe not as exciting). It's a chance to bond with your new baby in a way that goes beyond just weekends and evenings. Parental leave is about supporting your partner, sharing the load, and being an active part of those early days that are gone in the blink of an eye. You'll get to experience the ups and downs, the laughs and cries, and everything in between.

Gear Up

Preparing for parental leave as a first-time dad is like gearing up for the adventure of a lifetime. You're about to dive into a world of sleepless nights, baby giggles, and a whole lot of diaper changes. But before you take that leap, there's some planning to do. Think of it as getting your game plan ready.

- **Talk to Your Boss.** This might feel daunting, but preparation makes it smoother. Schedule a meeting well in advance of your expected leave date to talk about your plans. This shows your employer that you're proactive and considerate of the company's needs. Be transparent about your intentions and expected outcomes, and approach the conversation with a mindset of mutual benefit. This honest dialogue can foster understanding, ensuring both parties are on the same page.

- **Set Up Your Work Handover.** This can feel like passing the baton in a relay race - you want to make sure you tie up all loose ends to fully immerse yourself in baby bliss. Create a detailed plan of your responsibilities. Write a detailed handover document covering all the essential info, from ongoing projects to key contacts. This way, you can head off to diaper duty, knowing your work is covered and your coworkers won't be left hanging.

- **Keep in touch.** Stay in the loop if you can. This tends to make the transition smoother for everyone involved. It's all about striking a balance – the occasional quick check-in with your team to help keep things running smoothly at work while ensuring that you're present for your baby and partner, which is your number one priority. That way, you can enjoy your time off without feeling entirely out of the loop.

So, chat with your boss, plan ahead, and make sure things are in place for when you're away. Trust me, work will still be there when you return, but these early moments with your baby are priceless.

Make the Most of Your Time Off

Now that you've finally taken the plunge and scored some well-deserved time off for your new role as a dad, it's time for the fun part: making the most of it. This is your chance to dive into dadhood headfirst.

- **Be Present.** Take your mind off emails and deadlines and fully immerse yourself in family life. Focus on those little moments that'll make all the sleepless nights worth it.

- **Embrace the Chaos.** Dadhood can sometimes be messy and unpredictable, but that's part of the adventure. Enjoy every moment, and I mean every single moment.

- **Build Memories.** Whether it's that first wobbly attempt at tummy time, early morning snuggles, daily walks, reading bedtime stories, or simply rocking your baby to sleep, every moment is a priceless memory in the making. So, soak in the giggles and snap a million photos because these days will fly by faster than you think.

The Return

Returning to work after your first stint as a new dad can be a bit tricky. You've been knee-deep in diapers, midnight feedings, and the pure joy of baby giggles, and now it's time to navigate the world of deadlines and meetings again. Here's the deal: you've got this.

- **Ease back in.** Where possible, arrange a gradual return, maybe starting with a few half-days or remote work days, which, thanks to Covid, is a lot more straightforward nowadays. This will give you a chance to adjust without feeling overwhelmed. Keep in mind it's totally normal to miss your baby and feel a bit out of the loop. Stay connected with your family through quick video calls or photos throughout the day. Some days might feel like a breeze, while others could be a whirlwind. That's okay.

- **Stay flexible.** Finding the balance between returning to work and dadhood can be a juggling act, and you need to be flexible. You might find that your schedule needs some adjusting as every day won't go as planned, and that's alright. Some mornings might start with a baby meltdown, and you'll need to roll with the punches. Talk openly to your boss and colleagues about your needs, and don't be afraid to prioritise family time when necessary. Staying adaptable will help you manage both worlds more smoothly and make the transition back to work easier.

- **Continue bonding.** Just because you're back at work doesn't mean you have to miss out on bonding with your little one. Whether it's a morning cuddle before you head out or a bedtime story after a long day, these moments are gold. Keep up with those bonding routines you started during your leave - they can be a comforting constant for both you and your child. Remember, it's the quality time, not just the quantity, that counts. So, keep finding ways to connect, and you'll keep that bond strong, even with a busy schedule.

Returning to work can be a mixed bag of emotions – you're

excited to get back to the swing of things, yet a part of you misses those quiet moments with your little one. But, with some planning and flexibility, you can tackle this new chapter confidently.

In Conclusion

Mastering the juggle between work and dadhood is less about achieving a perfect balance and more about finding your rhythm. Even though it's a wild ride, every twist and turn will help you grow. Keep prioritising what truly matters, stay flexible, and don't forget to pat yourself on the back for even the smallest victories. You're not just surviving this juggle; you're mastering it, one step at a time, proving that dadhood and work can coexist harmoniously. So, take a deep breath, enjoy the moments, and keep being the amazing dad and professional you are.

From office to nursery, you're on the go,
Balancing meetings while the milk feeds flow.
Emails and burp cloths, a tightrope walk,
Whispering lullabies between Teams talks.

Coffee in hand, bags under eyes,
But every little smile makes the tiredness fly.
Laptop in one hand, baby in the other,
You're a multitasking dad: superhero undercover.

Late-night work sessions, rocking the crib,
Juggling both worlds, but never a fib.
With love and dedication, you conquer the day,
Dad, you've got this, come what may!

~ akin.o ~

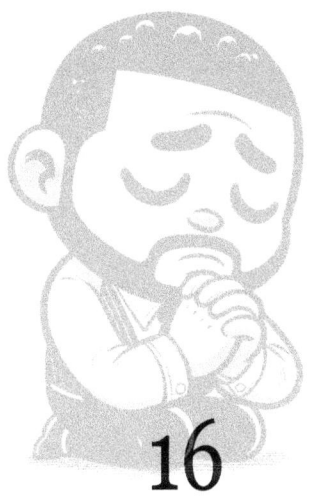

16

Faith-Filled Dadhood
The God Factor

Now, here's something that's deeper than dadhood itself - your relationship with God. The dadhood journey is full of divine moments, and your faith in God can be a solid foundation as you navigate the joys and challenges of raising your little one.

A New Dimension

Being a Christian adds a whole new dimension to this exciting adventure, as you'll find strength, inspiration and guidance through the highs and lows of being a dad. So, let's delve into how your faith can help you raise that incredible little creature with love, wisdom, and compassion.

Embracing God's Love

The cornerstone of Christianity is love, and there's no better place to start than by embracing and sharing God's love with your baby. From watching those tiny fingers curl around yours to those very first moments - hearing their first giggles, taking those first wobbly steps, and uttering their first "Dada" - let your child feel the warmth and security of unconditional love. Ephesians 3:17-19 reminds us to be rooted and grounded in love, and that's exactly what your baby needs. Show them they are cherished, valued and loved. Embracing God's love as a dad means blending patience, kindness, and endless support into every moment, knowing that no matter how many sleepless nights or diaper changes you face, God's walking by your side on this beautiful journey.

Building a Strong Spiritual Foundation

As a Christian dad, one of your most important roles is laying down the roots for a strong spiritual foundation for your little one. Embedding Christian values in everyday moments can transform the mundane into meaningful, faith-building experiences. Whether it's saying a quick prayer before bedtime, sharing Bible stories during storytime, singing Christian lullabies or embodying Christ's love and patience in your actions, it all adds to the nourishing of a budding spirit. Proverbs 22:6 reminds us: "Train up a child in the way he should go; even when he is old, he will not depart from it." By building this strong spiritual foundation, you're not just raising a child - you're nurturing a soul rooted in eternal love and guiding them through life's ups and downs with faith as their anchor.

Leading by Example

Babies are incredibly observant, even before they can speak. They watch and learn from your actions and attitudes, which reflect your beliefs and values. Whether by demonstrating love and forgiveness, showing kindness to others, practising patience, or being honest and fair - your baby will eventually pick up on these cues. James 1:22 says, "But be doers of the word, and not hearers only, deceiving yourselves." By living out your Christian values, you're setting a powerful example for your child to follow, teaching them not just through lessons but through a living testimony of God's love and grace in action. Your daily actions are the greatest sermon they'll ever witness.

Finding Comfort in Scripture

Being a dad comes with its own fair share of uncertainty, but turning to Scripture can provide all the comfort and guidance you need. Those moments when you feel overwhelmed, flip open the Bible and find a verse that speaks right to your heart. Isaiah 41:10 is a gem: "Fear not, for I am with you; be not dismayed, for I am your God; I will strengthen you, I will help you, I will uphold you with my righteous right hand." These words can be a soothing balm, reminding you that you're never truly alone on this journey. So, when you're facing sleepless nights, a colicky baby, or just the everyday challenges of dadhood, find solace in God's word and know you're not alone. Remember, being guided by the Word of God not only brings you peace but also sets a beautiful example for your little one.

Finding Purpose and Direction

It goes without saying that dadhood is filled with countless decisions and responsibilities. It can sometimes feel like embarking on a trip without a map - exciting yet sometimes a bit daunting. This is where your faith truly shines, offering a compass of purpose and direction. Raising your little one while anchored in faith helps you see the bigger picture: your role as a guide, protector, and teacher. Verses like Jeremiah 29:11, "For I know the plans I have for you, declares the Lord, plans for welfare and not for evil, to give you a future and a hope," can serve as a beacon during uncertain times. Knowing that God has a plan can provide peace, confidence, and an assurance that your tiny tot has a God-given path filled with love, faith, and endless possibilities.

The Power of Prayer

One of the most powerful tools in your dadhood toolkit is prayer. It's like a direct line to God. Pray for your baby's health, happiness, and future. Pray for wisdom and patience for yourself as you navigate dadhood. Remember, when you pray for your baby, you're not just speaking words into the air - you're inviting God's presence and protection over your little one. Philippians 4:6-7 reminds us: "Do not be anxious about anything, but in every situation, by prayer and petition, with thanksgiving, present your requests to God. And the peace of God, which transcends all understanding, will guard your hearts and your minds in Christ Jesus." Embracing the power of prayer as a dad brings comfort and direction, showing your child that no matter what life throws their way, there's always a divine shoulder to lean on. Make prayer a daily habit, and as your child grows, encourage them to pray as well. It's a beautiful way to build a strong spiritual connection and teach them the importance of communicating with God.

Celebrating Faith in Milestones and Everyday Life

Celebrating milestones - big or small - and the everyday moments that make up your baby's life are the joys of being a dad. When you incorporate your faith, these celebrations become even more meaningful. Whether it's your baby's first steps, their first birthday, or just a simple cuddle on the couch, take a moment to thank God for these precious gifts. Colossians 3:17 reminds us: "And whatever you do, whether in word or deed, do it all in the name of the Lord Jesus, giving thanks to God the Father through him." By infusing faith into these moments, you're not just celebrating your child's growth - you're acknowledging the grace and blessings from God that make these moments possible. It's about cherishing every day, finding joy in the little things, and teaching your child to see God's hand in every aspect of life.

Instilling Biblical Values

Dadhood is an incredible responsibility, especially when it comes to instilling values in your little one. Your faith adds a beautiful depth to this task, providing a foundation of love, kindness, and integrity. Imagine teaching your child the importance of honesty by sharing stories from the Bible or showing them the power of compassion through everyday acts of kindness. Verses like Galatians 5:22-23, which talk about the fruits of the Spirit - love, joy, peace, patience, kindness, goodness, faithfulness, gentleness, and self-control - serve as a wonderful guide. By living out these values yourself, you're not just telling your child what's important; you're showing them through your actions.

Finding Community Support

Sometimes, you can feel like you're juggling a million things at once and finding community support can make a big difference. Getting involved in your local church, parenting groups, or community activities can connect you with other dads walking similar paths. Surround yourself with those who share your faith and offer encouragement, practical advice, spiritual support, friendship and a sense of belonging. Hebrews 10:24-25 reminds us: "And let us consider how we may spur one another on toward love and good deeds, not giving up meeting together, as some are in the habit of doing, but encouraging one another." By leaning into this support, you're building a network of faith-filled friends who uplift and inspire each other through the ups and downs of dadhood. Also, over time, it's an excellent way for your child to make friends and grow their own faith.

Embracing Grace and Forgiveness

Dadhood is a journey full of learning curves; sometimes, you'll make mistakes. That's why it's crucial to embrace forgiveness and grace. There will be times when you lose your cool or feel overwhelmed, and that's okay. What truly matters is how you handle these moments. Let's take a leaf out of Ephesians 4:32: "Be kind and compassionate to one another, forgiving each other, just as in Christ God forgave you." When things don't go as planned, remember to seek forgiveness and start afresh. Teach your little one that it's okay to stumble as long as they get back up with a heart full of grace. This creates a loving and forgiving environment where your child feels safe and understood.

Encouraging Spiritual Growth
As your baby gradually becomes a curious toddler and beyond, encourage their spiritual growth. Motivate them with age-appropriate resources such as children's Bibles, Christian books, music, and activities. Take them to Sunday school and get them involved in youth group activities. Answer their questions about faith with honesty and enthusiasm. By feeding their spiritual curiosity and weaving faith into the fabric of daily life, you're planting seeds of spirituality that will grow and flourish as your child matures. It's all about making faith a natural part of their world, showing them that God's love and guidance are always there to lean on, no matter what life brings. You're also helping them build a personal relationship with God that will guide them all through their lives.

Words of Wisdom

Though the beautiful whirlwind of dadhood may have its ups and downs, with faith as your anchor, every step you take will be infused with meaning and divine joy. From leading by example to encouraging spiritual growth, your faith can be a powerful and positive force in your role as a dad. So, embrace it, share it, and let it shine through every moment. Remember God's promise in Proverbs 22:6: "Train up a child in the way he should go; even when he is old, he will not depart from it." Your prayer should simply be for God to give you the wisdom, knowledge and understanding to train your child the right way, and with each passed-down faith lesson, you can rest assured that your little one is becoming who God destined them to be.

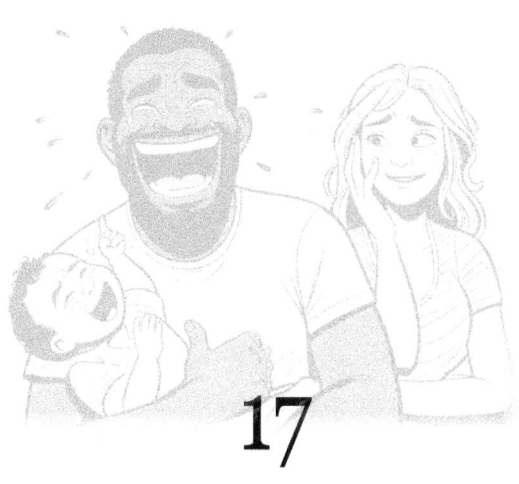

17

Laughing Through Dadhood
Dad Jokes

Becoming a dad comes with its own special perk: the license to tell the cheesiest, corniest, groan-inducing, eye-rolling jokes that somehow manage to brighten even the toughest of days. But, they're not just for cheap laughs or embarrassing your kids in public; they're the unsung heroes of dadhood!

A Touch of Magic

Dad jokes can turn a meltdown into a moment of connection and transform exhaustion into a shared chuckle. They're also, in my opinion, one of the secret ingredients needed to help master the fine art of being an awesome dad. Here are some things you should know about this "hidden" gem.

It's Free!
Let's face it, parenting can be tough. It's like a 24/7 job with no vacation, and the pay is...well, let's not talk about that.

But laughter? Laughter is free. It's been scientifically proven to alleviate stress and strengthen family bonds, making it one of the most effective tools in your dadhood arsenal. According to a study published in PLOS One, children raised with humour report better relationships with their parents and are more likely to use similar techniques in their own parenting. So, first-time dad, when life hands you a toddler tantrum or a baby blowout, remember this: a good laugh can diffuse tension, foster connection, and even help with creative problem-solving. Plus, it's a lot cheaper than therapy.

The Ultimate Icebreaker

Classic dad jokes are the cornerstone of dadhood, a rite of passage if you will. They're the ultimate icebreaker, capable of eliciting eye rolls and groans in equal measure. But why do they continue to be a staple in the dad toolkit? Perhaps it's because they serve as a reminder that not everything has to be serious. In the words of a joke from Today.com, "What did the beach say when the tide came in? Long time no sea". It's simple, corny, and guaranteed to get at least a chuckle, even if it's out of pity. The beauty of dad jokes lies in their simplicity. They don't require a setup or a punchline that takes three paragraphs to deliver. They're quick, effective, and a great way to lighten the mood. Crafting your own dad jokes is an art form. Start with a basic pun or play on words, and let your imagination do the rest. Remember, the key is not to take yourself too seriously. After all, it's the groan-induced laughter that makes them memorable.

Turning Oops into Laughs

Let's be honest: parenting is a masterclass in humility, often taught through the medium of epic failures. It's like being handed a test for which you're only partially prepared, and the questions keep changing. But here's the thing: those parenting fails are comedy gold! They're the stories you'll tell over and over, each time with a little more embellishment and a lot more laughter. Take the classic diaper mishap, for instance. You're in the middle of changing a diaper when your little one decides to demonstrate their newfound ability to pee like a fountain. It's a rite of passage, a moment that teaches you the importance of speed and precision. And then there are the misunderstood baby cues. You think they want to play, but really, they're just hungry. Again. These moments are not just mistakes; they're memories in the making that you'll look back on and laugh about for years to come.

Humour in Mess and Chaos

I know I already said this, but dadhood is packed with unexpected twists and turns, each more unpredictable than the last. One moment, you're enjoying a peaceful meal, and the next, you're wearing it. Kids have an uncanny ability to turn mealtime into a Jackson Pollock painting, leaving you wondering how they managed to get spaghetti sauce in places that defy physics. But in those messy moments, there's a certain beauty. It's the realisation that life is messy, too, and that's okay. Then there's the classic miscommunication with your partner, where you're convinced they said "wipers" when they actually meant "diapers." It's in these moments of confusion and chaos that you find the humour, the shared laughter that reminds you that you're both in this together.

Turning Challenges into Comedy

Challenges are par for the course in dadhood, but with a bit of humour, they can become opportunities for connection. Take tantrums, for example. They're loud, they're dramatic, and they're utterly exhausting. But they're also a part of life with young children. Instead of viewing them as disasters, try reframing them as scenes from a comedy. Imagine narrating your child's tantrum like a sports commentator, complete with play-by-play analysis. It doesn't change the fact that you're dealing with a meltdown, but it does shift your perspective, allowing you to see the humour in the situation. And those late-night wake-up calls? They're prime opportunities for finding joy. When you're up at 3 a.m., rocking a baby back to sleep, take a moment to appreciate the quiet, the stillness, and the soft glow of the nightlight. These are the moments that pass all too quickly, and finding joy in them can make the journey all the more rewarding.

Laughing Through the Imperfections
A light-hearted perspective is a gift you give yourself. It's about accepting that not everything needs to be perfect. That life is full of imperfections, and that's what makes it interesting. Embrace the unexpected, the bumps in the road that make the journey worthwhile. It's about laughing at the chaos and seeing the humour in the everyday struggles that come with dadhood. In doing so, you'll find that the journey becomes a little less daunting and a lot more enjoyable. Laughter is not just an escape from the challenges; it's a way to embrace them and find joy in the midst of the storm.

Turning Lessons into Playful Adventures
Humour is a powerful teaching tool that can make lessons memorable and engaging for children. Imagine trying to teach your child about safety rules, but instead of a stern lecture, you turn it into a playful scenario. When you sprinkle in a few dad jokes, you transform chores and rules into light-hearted moments that stick. Teaching about kindness? Use a joke to illustrate the point. Perhaps you're role-playing with stuffed animals, demonstrating the importance of looking both ways before crossing the street. Cleaning up toys? Make it an entertaining game, complete with funny rewards for a job well done. It's all about showing that learning can be fun, about showing your child that life is full of lessons, but those lessons don't have to be boring. By using humour, you're not just teaching your child; you're also building a bond, creating a shared experience that both of you will treasure forever.

The Ultimate Stress-Buster
Laughter is a remarkable thing. It's a stress-relief technique that's available to everyone, regardless of age or circumstance.

It's been shown to reduce stress hormones like epinephrine and cortisol while boosting mood-elevating chemicals like dopamine and serotonin. In the world of parenting, where stress is a constant companion, laughter offers a welcome reprieve. It builds emotional resilience, not just for you but for your children as well. It teaches them that life has its ups and downs, but laughter is a constant. Encouraging laughter as a family tradition fosters an environment of joy and connection, creating memories that last a lifetime.

Creating Family Traditions
Dad jokes are more than just a collection of cheesy one-liners – they're a way to create lasting family traditions. Over time, it's not just about the jokes but the shared laughs and the memories that stick. Whether it's the classic "What do you call two monkeys that share an Amazon account? Prime mates!" a homemade pun, a funny story at dinner or a shared memory before bedtime, these moments of humour bring everyone closer. By making dad jokes a regular part of your family life, you're not just entertaining the kids - you're building a legacy of laughter and connection that will be cherished for years to come. Creating a family tradition of laughter and sharing daily funny moments helps maintain a positive outlook. It builds a foundation of happiness and resilience and creates lasting memories that bring everyone together with a laugh. They remind you that no matter how chaotic life gets, there's always room for a good dose of humour.

The Sweet Melody of Laughter

In the grand tapestry of dadhood, laughter is the thread that weaves it all together. It's the melody that plays in the background, a constant reminder that life is full of surprises, and it's all the more beautiful for it. As you navigate the challenges and joys of dadhood, let laughter be your guide, your companion on this incredible adventure. Find joy in the unexpected, embrace the chaos and remember that through it all, laughter is one of the greatest gifts you can give yourself and your family.

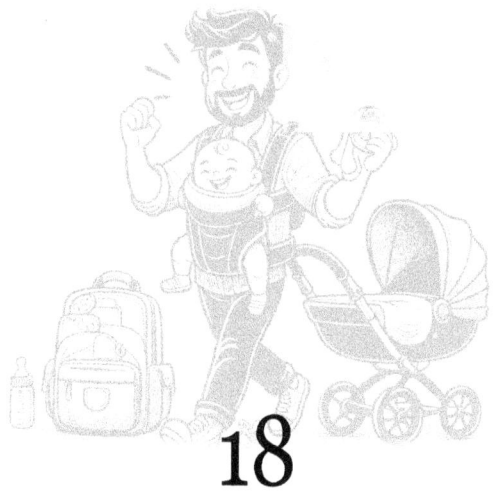

18

Must-Haves for New Dads
The Complete Toolkit

If you're feeling a mix of excitement and nerves, you're right where you need to be. As you've heard me say in more ways than one, dadhood is an incredible journey full of unforgettable moments, but having the right tools can make this wild ride even more enjoyable. From essential gear to handy tech, insightful books, and the emotional stuff, the paragraphs you're about to read are your go-to resource when navigating the exciting adventure of being a dad with confidence and a bit of flair.

The Essential Gear Toolkit

When it comes to being a first-time dad, having the right essentials can make your life a whole lot easier. Think of it as your superpower kit - everything you need to make your life as a new dad as smooth as silk.

The Must-Haves and Nice-To-Haves

- **Diaper Bag.** A good diaper bag is like a portable command centre - keeping all your baby essentials organised and within reach. I'd opt for one with multiple compartments and pockets so you can easily find that pacifier or extra pair of socks when you need them most. It might also be a good idea to choose one that's not only functional but stylish too because you'll be carrying it around a lot!

- **Diapers, Wipes, and Creams.** These are the holy trinity of baby care. Diapers keep your baby dry and comfy, wipes are perfect for quick cleanups, and creams help prevent and soothe diaper rashes. Stock up on these essentials because you'll go through them at the speed of light! A well-stocked supply means you're always ready for those unexpected poop leaks and can keep your baby happy and rash-free.

- **Pacifiers.** These are handy for calming your fussy baby and helping them doze off. Look for one that's easy to clean and made from safe, BPA-free materials. Having a few pacifiers on hand means you're always prepared for those moments when your little one needs a bit of extra comfort. They can also be a helpful tool for keeping your little one occupied while you tackle other tasks.

- **Bottle Warmer.** This is a lifesaver for those middle-of-the-night feeds. Look for one that's easy to use and heats evenly. Trust me, having a bottle warmer in your toolkit will make those midnight feedings much more straightforward and give you a bit more shut-eye time.

- **Changing Mat.** Whether at home or out and about, having a reliable changing mat means you're always prepared for those unexpected diaper blowouts. Grab one that's portable, practical, easy to clean and has a waterproof surface to keep things mess-free.

- **Swaddle Blankets.** These are like magic hugs that help your baby feel secure and cosy, mimicking the snug environment of the womb. They calm a fussy baby and reduce the startle reflex, giving you some much-needed peace and quiet. They can double as burp cloths or blankets, so you'll get plenty of use out of them. Look for swaddles that are soft, lightweight, and easy to use.

- **Baby Carrier.** Perfect for keeping your hands free while keeping your baby close. Whether you're trying to soothe your baby to sleep or need to get stuff done around the house, a good baby carrier can be a game-changer. Look for one with good back support and adjustable straps for maximum comfort. Not only does it make life easier, but it also gives you that precious bonding time with your tiny tot.

- **Baby Clothes.** Choosing the right baby clothes is all about comfort and convenience. Look for soft, breathable fabrics that are gentle on your baby's skin. Onesies with snap buttons are ideal for quick changes, and having a variety of sizes on hand means you're always prepared for growth spurts. And don't forget the cute hats and socks to keep your baby cosy.

- **The Play Gym.** These colourful, interactive setups often come with hanging toys, mirrors, and soft mats that encourage your baby to reach, grab, and explore. Not only do they provide endless fun, but they also help with your baby's development by promoting motor skills and sensory exploration. Plus, it gives you a few moments to catch your breath while your baby is happily occupied.

- **Inflatable Bath Set.** They often come with cute designs and built-in toys and are a safe, fun, and easy-to-clean environment for your little one. Plus, they're portable, so you can set them up anywhere - perfect for those impromptu baths. Having an inflatable bath set means bath time becomes a playful and enjoyable experience for you and your baby.

- **Swing or Bouncer.** While swings gently rock your baby back and forth, bouncers provide a safe place for them to jump and wiggle. Both options are perfect for keeping your little one entertained and soothing them when they're fussy. They're handy when you need a few moments to catch your breath or get something done around the house. They're also great for helping your baby develop their motor skills and balance.

Well, I'll leave what qualifies as a must-have or nice-to-have up to you, but with these items in your arsenal, you'll be well-prepared to handle anything that comes your way. Remember, it's all about making your life a little easier and keeping your baby happy and comfortable.

The Tech Toolkit

In this digital age, there's a plethora of tech gadgets that can make dadhood a bit easier. From baby monitors to smart thermometers, tech can keep your little one safe and happy. It's time to embrace your inner geek and make parenting more high-tech!

- **Baby Monitor.** A good baby monitor with video and audio capabilities lets you keep an eye (and ear) on your little one from anywhere in the house without disturbing their sleep. Some even come with features like temperature monitoring and night vision. Having a reliable baby monitor means you can relax a bit more, knowing you're always connected to your baby.

- **White Noise Machine.** These handy gadgets create soothing, ambient sounds that help calm your baby and lull them to sleep. Look for one with different sound options so you can find the perfect one for your baby. They're great for drowning out background noise and creating a consistent, comforting sleep environment. They can also help you get that much-needed rest.

- **Smart Thermometer.** These nifty gadgets make taking your baby's temperature quick and easy, giving you accurate readings in seconds. Many smart thermometers can sync with your phone, track temperature trends, and even remind you when to take another reading. Having one of these in your toolkit means you can keep a close eye on your little one's health with minimal fuss.

- **Smart Home Devices.** These gadgets can do everything from turning your lights on to adjusting the thermostat, all with a tap on your phone or a simple voice command - super handy when your hands are full. You can check on your baby with a smart camera, control the baby monitor, or even play lullabies with a smart speaker. Smart home devices help create a more comfortable and convenient environment for you and your family.

- **Parenting Apps.** These apps can help you track feedings, diaper changes, sleep schedules, and even your baby's milestones. Some offer helpful tips and advice, connect you with other parents, and provide resources for everything from baby health to meal planning. With a good parenting app, you'll have all the information you need right at your fingertips. Here are a few apps to consider:

    ◦ **Baby Tracker.** Offers a simple, streamlined way to track feeding, diaper changes, sleep, and growth milestones.

    ◦ **WebMD Baby.** Provides information on infant care, including health, development, and common concerns during the first year.

- ○ **Cozi Family Organiser.** Shares calendars, custody schedules, recipes, grocery lists, tasks, and notes. It keeps all your lists and schedules in one place.

- ○ **AppClose.** Allows users to manage schedules, track expenses, send & receive money for reimbursement obligations and send date-stamped messages.

- ○ **Baby Connect.** Helps parents and caretakers track a baby's development and share information with relevant third parties such as physicians, caseworkers, family members, or babysitters.

- ○ **The Wonder Weeks.** a baby app that provides information about a baby's mental development through "leaps". It also helps parents understand why their baby is crying or acting differently and what they can do to help.

Embracing technology can make dadhood a lot more fun. So, keep exploring, stay curious, and enjoy raising your little one with a touch of tech magic.

The "Must-Reads" Toolkit

Whether you're looking for practical advice, heartwarming stories, or a good laugh, there's a book for every dad. Here are just a few reads that offer valuable insights, tips, and inspiration to help navigate dadhood:

- **"The Expectant Father" by Armin A. Brott and Jennifer Ash.** A comprehensive guide offering practical advice, tips, and emotional support to help fathers navigate everything from pregnancy to childbirth.

- **"Dude, You're Gonna Be a Dad!" by John Pfeiffer.** A

humorous yet practical read that's perfect for first-time dads.

- **"How to Be a Great Dad" by Keith Zafren.** A heartfelt guide packed with practical advice and tips for dads who want to build strong, positive relationships with their children.

- **"Be Prepared: A Practical Handbook for New Dads" by Gary Greenberg and Jeannie Hayden.** A humorous and informative guide for new dads full of useful tips and tricks, with illustrations, helpful diagrams, and real-life anecdotes.

- **"The New Father. A Dad's Guide to the First Year" by Armin A. Brott:** An insightful month-by-month guide for new dads, focusing on the first year of fatherhood.

These books are packed with practical tips, heartfelt stories, and valuable advice to help you navigate your dadhood journey. So, grab a cosy reading spot, and get ready to be the best dad you can be.

The "Online Resources" Toolkit

The internet is a goldmine with resources, support, and community all at your fingertips. Whether you're looking for tips on baby care, connecting with other dads, or finding the best baby gear, there's a wealth of information out there to help you along the way. Here are some go-to websites and online communities that can make your parenting journey a little smoother and a lot more connected:

- **Dadvengers** *(dadvengers.com)*. A community that supports and empowers dads through resources, events, and a supportive network, helping them navigate the challenges and joys of parenthood

while promoting positive mental health.

- **BabyCenter** *(babycenter.com)*. A comprehensive online resource for parents and expecting parents, offering medically reviewed information on pregnancy, childbirth, and early childhood development. It provides expert advice, weekly newsletters, and a helpful community where parents can connect and share experiences.

- **BabyCentre** *(babycentre.co.uk)*. The UK version of BabyCenter

- **Fatherly** *(fatherly.com)*. This Offers a wealth of articles, tips, advice, product recommendations, and resources for dads at every stage. It also provides articles, videos, and podcasts to support dads on their parenting journey.

- **Reddit's r/daddit** *(reddit.com/r/daddit)*. A supportive online community where dads can ask questions, offer advice, and connect with other fathers.

- **National Responsible Fatherhood Clearinghouse** *(fatherhood.gov)*. Provides support, research and innovative strategies to encourage and strengthen fathers and families. It offers a variety of resources for fathers, practitioners, and programs aimed at promoting responsible fatherhood and healthy family relationships.

- **Dadsnet** *(dadsnet.com)*. An online community offering support, advice, and a sense of camaraderie among dads. It features articles, videos, podcasts, and forums where dads can connect, share experiences, and find helpful information.

The internet is brimming with resources to help you navigate dadhood. So, dive in, explore, and avail yourself of these useful digital tools. You won't regret it.

The Emotional Toolkit

As you already know, being a dad isn't just about the practical stuff; it's also about being emotionally present and supportive of your little one. This toolkit includes everything from patience and empathy to self-care and love.

- **Patience.** This is the virtue of parenthood. From late-night feedings to those epic diaper blowouts, being patient with your baby is key. It's all about taking a deep breath, staying calm, and understanding that your little one is learning and growing every day. Those tough moments won't last forever, and your patience will help create a loving and secure environment for your baby to thrive. So, hang in there and embrace the challenges; your patience will not only help you stay sane but ultimately teach your child the importance of staying calm under pressure.

- **Empathy.** This is all about tuning into your baby's feelings and experiences, even when they can't tell you what's wrong. When your newborn is fussy or crying, try to imagine what might be going on in their tiny world - maybe they're hungry, tired, or simply need a cuddle. By responding with love and understanding, you show your baby that their feelings matter and they're safe with you. It's a beautiful way to build trust and a loving emotional bond that will last a lifetime.

- **Sound Communication.** Even though your little one might not be able to form complete sentences yet, communication is still key. From those precious coos and babbles to the way they look at you with wide, curious eyes, your baby is always trying to communicate. Responding with smiles, gentle words, and soothing tones helps create a strong bond and lets your baby know they are understood and loved. Good communication sets the foundation for a lifetime of trust and connection, so keep the conversation flowing, no matter how tiny the words might be!

- **Sense of Humour.** Babies are full of surprises, and having a sense of humour can turn those unexpected moments into joyful memories. From silly faces and goofy voices to laughing at the little mishaps, humour helps you bond with your baby and keeps things light-hearted. Plus, laughter is contagious and creates a happy, positive environment for your little one to grow up in. So, tap into your inner comedian, enjoy the giggles, and let your sense of humour be the glue that brings you and your baby closer together!

- **Self-Care.** So often overlooked but incredibly important. Dadhood can be demanding, and it's easy to forget your own needs. But remember, a happy and healthy dad makes for a happy and healthy baby. Whether it's grabbing a few moments of quiet with your morning Horlicks, catching up on a hobby, or even just taking a nap when you can, self-care helps you recharge and be your best self for your little one. Remember, it's okay to take a break and look after yourself; self-care isn't being selfish! Your well-being is key to being the fantastic dad you want to be!

- **Flexibility.** Dadhood is full of surprises, and being flexible helps you roll with the punches. Plans might change, routines can get disrupted, and sometimes things don't go as expected. But embracing flexibility means being open to new approaches and adapting to your baby's ever-changing needs. It's about finding balance and making the best of every situation. So, loosen up, go with the flow, and let flexibility guide you through the twists and turns of dadhood.

- **Resilience.** Life as a dad can be full of challenges, but resilience is what helps you bounce back stronger every time. It's about staying positive, facing difficulties head-on, coming out stronger on the other side and finding solutions instead of dwelling on problems. By showing resilience, you will inspire your child to face their own challenges with courage and determination.

- **Love.** This is the foundation of your emotional toolkit! It's the driving force behind everything you do as a dad. Show your love through hugs, kisses, attention, and being there for your bundle of joy. Let your little one know they are cherished and valued every single day. Your love creates a secure, nurturing environment where your baby can thrive and grow. So, pour your heart into every moment.

Every moment with your little one is an opportunity to connect and grow on a deeper level. Keep the tools in this toolkit close, trust yourself, and tackle dadhood with confidence and heart. Remember, you've got all it takes to be an amazing dad!

Final Thoughts

So, there you have it, the first-time dad's complete toolkit. From the practical to the emotional, you're equipped with everything you need to tackle the challenges and cherish the joys of being a dad. Embrace the twists and turns, treasure the small moments, and let your heart lead the way. Remember, with the right tools, some patience, a sense of humour, a lot of love and a trust in God - if you're a person of faith – you'll shape your child's world in the most beautiful way.

We all know there's so much to acquire,
From gear to gadgets, and remember the pacifier.
A sturdy stroller for walks in the park,
And even a monitor to hear every bark.

Tech to capture those firsts in HD,
And an app to track your little one's sleep.
Books full of wisdom from dads who've been there,
With tips and tricks on how to best care.

Emotional support from family and friends,
Patience and love, which never ends.
With these must-haves, you're ready to go,
On the grand adventure of the Dadhood show.

~ akin.o ~

The Outro
It's Been Real!

Can you believe it? It feels like yesterday when you and your partner were staring at that positive pregnancy test. And now, look at you - armed with valuable knowledge, ready to tackle the world of dadhood with confidence and a wide smile. Let's take a moment to reflect on the journey we've been on.

We started this adventure by redefining fatherhood before diving into the wonderful chaos of preparing to be a dad. From understanding the stages of pregnancy and baby development to budgeting for baby essentials and mastering the art of assembling a cot without losing your sanity, you're gradually becoming an expert at anticipating the unexpected.

If you're still going through the trimesters, then I'm sure that with each passing day, you're learning what it takes to support your partner through the highs and lows of pregnancy and understanding that your role as a dad-to-be is mega important. And if you've already experienced the big push, I know beyond a shadow of a doubt that you were a real-life hero during labour and delivery, showing the importance of your presence by offering full-on support and maybe shedding a tear of joy while at it.

So, new dad, what's it like embracing the whirlwind of diaper changes, night feedings, baby cues, and sleepless nights? I get the feeling you're handling it like a pro. I've also got no doubts that you're continually prioritising your little one's health, baby-proofing your home, and building emotional bonds, not just with your baby but with your partner, too. All in all, it looks like you've got everything in hand.

However, this is just the beginning. Dadhood is a lifelong journey. Embrace your unique parenting style - remember, you're one of a kind! Don't take your relationship with your partner for granted - keep speaking each other's love languages and fanning the flames of romance amidst the chaos. Be grateful for every milestone and keep the humour alive with those dad jokes – you'll be surprised at how they can turn the most challenging moments into opportunities for laughter. And, here's one I can't emphasise enough - through the hustle and bustle of life, make sure you take good care of yourself. Remember, healthy dad, healthy family!

Keep exploring the resources we've talked about. There's always something new to learn. Revisit chapters when you need a refresher, and don't hesitate to apply your newly acquired insights to your everyday life. Keep an open mind to new experiences and be excited to seek out new knowledge and support. Every bit of wisdom you gather will make you an even better dad.

Remember, you're not just making it through dadhood - you're thriving! Your role as a dad is powerful and transformative. You have the strength, adaptability, and love to make a meaningful impact in your child's life, and if you're a man of faith, you've got the God factor, too. So, approach dadhood with a sense of adventure and fulfilment, knowing that you're shaping the future, one prayer, one bedtime story and one diaper change at a time.

So, from the bottom of my heart, thank you for joining me on this incredible journey. Your commitment to becoming the best dad you can be is truly inspiring. I hope this book will continue to be a source of support and laughter as you navigate the joys and challenges of dadhood. Here's to you

The Outro

and the exciting journey ahead - make it a memorable one!

This guide is written, the last word penned,
But your dadhood story will never end.
Each day ahead, a page anew,
A life to shape, a world to view.

From first-time fears to moments of pride,
You've learned to lead, to love, to guide.
Through chaos, calm, the highs and lows,
Your dad-heart forever grows.

Through every challenge, each small success,
You've turned uncertainty into progress.
For it's not perfection that makes you great,
But the love you give - the dad you create.

The tears, the laughter, the moments shared,
Each one a bond that says, "You care."
Dadhood's not a script, nor is it a chart,
It's a lifetime role played by the heart.

So, though this book may conclude its tale,
Your dad-heart will never fail.
This guide is merely the starting line,
The rest of the story is yours to define.

For no map can plot what's uniquely yours,
With laughter and love, stay the course.
Continue the journey with a can-do attitude,
And remember, to your child,
THE BESTEST DAD IS YOU!

~ akin.o ~

Acknowledgements

I believe every journey worth taking is one led by The Almighty and shared with the people who walk beside you, cheer you on, and pick you up when you stumble. Writing this book has been no different. There are so many people to thank for helping bring *"The Essential Guide for First-Time Dads"* to life, and this page is dedicated to you.

To the Beginning and the End. Thank You for inspiring the words on these pages and giving me the patience, clarity, and courage to share this message with others. Without Your presence, this book wouldn't have seen the light of day.

To my dear wife, Debs. You've been my rock, my sounding board, and my endless source of inspiration. Your love, patience, unwavering support, and belief in me made this book and my journey into dadhood possible. With you, parenting is an exciting team sport, and I'm so glad we're in it together.

My darling angels, Oyindamolaoluwa and Oluwatishe. You're the God-given gifts who sparked this adventure! Thank you for teaching me what it truly means to be a dad and making me the dad I am today. Every smile, giggle, tear, sleepless night, and chaotic moment has been a lesson in unconditional love, patience, and finding joy in the unexpected. You've taught me lessons no book ever could and given me stories worth sharing. You truly are my inspiration in every sense of the word. And thank you for letting me use your cushion *(wink, wink!)*

And, of course, my sibs! Ever dependable, ever reliable. I know the Good Book talks about a friend that sticks closer than a brother, but with you guys in my life, a friend like that will almost be impossible to find. I'm blessed to have y'all!

To an incredible friend and mentor, Bajo Akisanya (Pastor). My special thanks go out to you for graciously taking on the challenge of writing the foreword for this book. Your words set the tone perfectly, blending wisdom and heart in a way only you can. Your encouragement and friendship are gifts I'll always treasure. Thank you!

To my friend, Bola Balogun. You sparked, in part, the inspiration for this book in a way you may not even realise. Thank you for reminding me of the impact that honest, relatable, and heartfelt advice can have in guiding new dads through one of life's greatest adventures. This book is a testament to the inspiration you've given me, and I'm grateful to have had your influence on this journey.

To all the dads, and dads-to-be, out there. One could say that this book wouldn't exist without you. Your shared experiences, questions, stories and even your dad jokes have fuelled the pages of this book. You reminded me that no two dad journeys are the same, but we all share a determination to give our kids the best we can. So, this one's for you!

A big shout-out to the creatives, too. You brought humour and heart to this project, and your creativity has added a spark that words alone could never do. Thank you for bringing these pages to life.

And finally, to you, the reader. Whether you're a new dad, a dad-to-be, or someone looking to understand and support the dads in your life, thank you for picking up this guide and deciding to dive in. Thank you for trusting me to be a part of your journey. I hope this book brings you a laugh when you need it, a tip to make life easier, and the confidence to know you've got this.

Here's to dadhood, the greatest adventure of all time!

About Akin

Akin Olunloyo is a passionate father, husband, and advocate for all things fatherhood. With over two decades of experience in parenting, Akin has a genuine love for helping new dads navigate the various stages of fatherhood.

A proud father of two daughters, Akin knows the challenges and joys of raising children. He has spent countless hours reading bedtime stories, changing diapers, and soothing midnight tears, all while maintaining a thriving, healthy work-life balance. His personal journey through fatherhood has inspired him to share his insights, tips, and heartfelt advice with other dads and dads-to-be.

Akin's writing is characterised by its informal and relatable tone with a touch of humour. He believes that laughter is essential to parenting and that every dad can find their unique way to shine. His goal is to empower fathers to embrace their role with confidence, compassion, and a sense of adventure and to also remind them that they're not alone on this journey.

His book, *The Essential Guide for First-Time Dads*, is a culmination of his experiences, research, and conversations with other dads who have walked the same path.

Akin is an active member of a men's mentoring group, a singer/songwriter, and enjoys spending quality time with his family, perfecting his dad jokes. He resides in the UK with his wife and two daughters.

You can catch up with Akin on...

Instagram: @Dadhood_Unplugged
Facebook: @DadhoodUnplugged

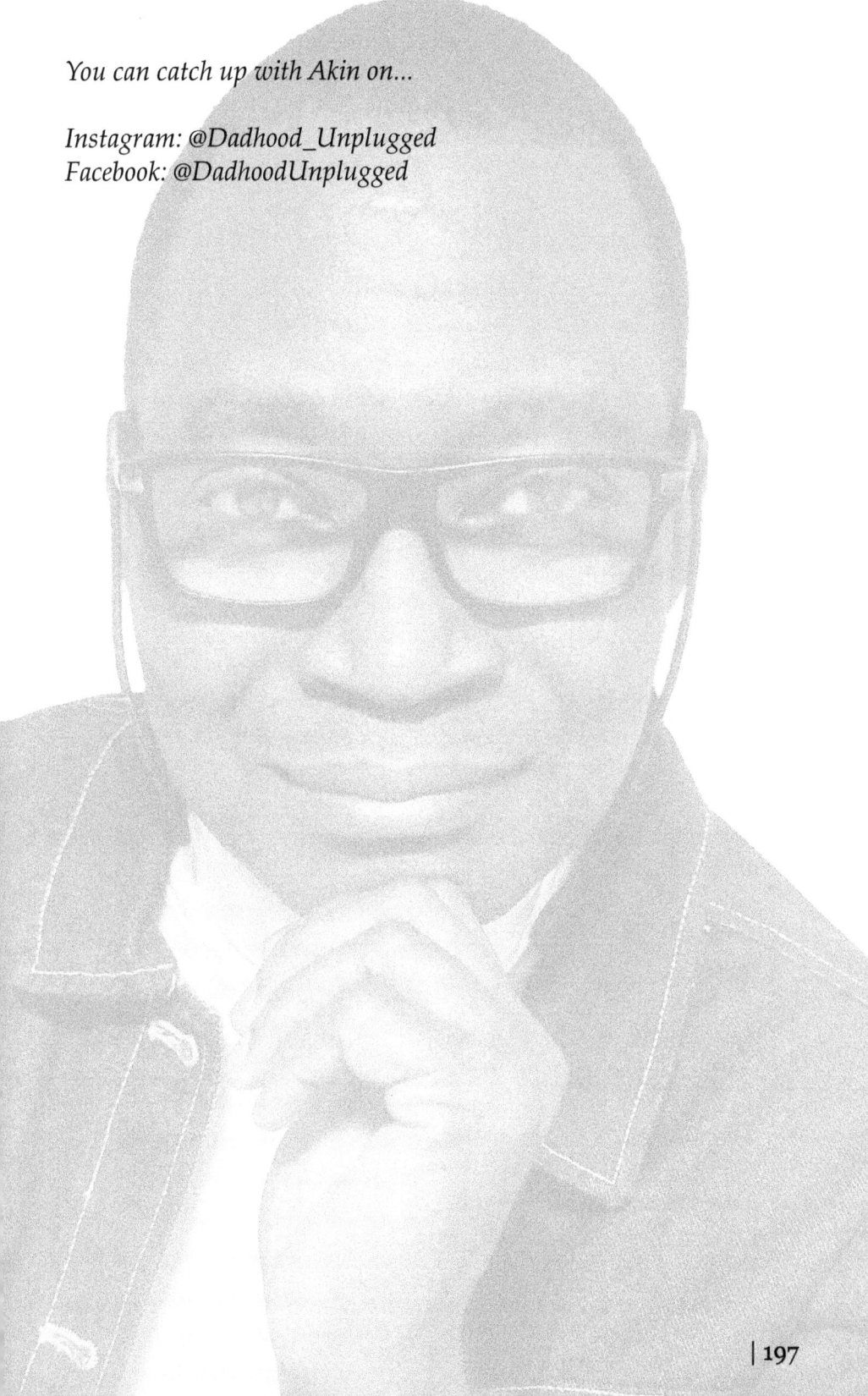

Glossary

Welcome to your go-to guide to help you make sense of all the medical jargon, parenting lingo, developmental milestones and feeding and nutrition vocab you'll encounter as you embark on this exciting journey.

Medical Jargon

- **Alpha-fetoprotein (AFP).** A protein produced by the foetus.

- **Amniocentesis.** A prenatal test that involves extracting a small amount of amniotic fluid from a pregnant woman's uterus to check for genetic abnormalities.

- **Amniotic fluid.** The liquid that surrounds your baby in the uterus (also called "waters").

- **Amniotic sac.** A thin-walled sac that surrounds the baby inside the uterus.

- **Anaesthetic.** A drug that causes total or partial loss of sensation in a part or the whole of the body.

- **Anaesthetist.** A doctor who specialises in giving anaesthetic.

- **Anaphylaxis.** A severe and potentially life-threatening allergic reaction that needs immediate treatment.

- **Anomaly scan.** A detailed ultrasound scan offered between 18 and 21 weeks of pregnancy to check for physical conditions that may affect your baby.

- **Antenatal.** A term that means "before birth" (alternative terms are "prenatal" and "antepartum").

- **Apgar score.** A test given one minute after your baby is born, then again 5 minutes later, that assesses a baby's appearance (skin colour), pulse, grimace (reflex), activity (muscle tone) and respiration. A perfect Apgar score is 10; typical Apgar scores are 7, 8 or 9. A score lower than 7 means that your baby might need help breathing.

- **Baby waters.** The amniotic fluid that surrounds and protects a baby in the womb.

- **Birth plan.** A written document describing your partner's preferences for her care during labour and birth.

- **Braxton Hicks contractions.** Mild, irregular uterine contractions that occur during pregnancy, often described as "practice contractions" or "false labour" because they are the body's way of preparing for real labour but do not signify that labour has started; they usually feel like a tightening sensation in the abdomen and are generally not painful.

- **Breech.** When the baby is positioned inside the uterus with its bottom or feet down instead of its head.

- **Caesarean section.** A surgical procedure in which a baby is delivered through a cut in the abdomen and uterus (also called a "C-section").

- **Cervix.** The narrow, lower end of the uterus that softens and opens during labour to allow your baby to come out.

- **Colic.** A condition in which a healthy baby cries for long periods of time for no obvious reason.

- **Colostrum.** The first breast milk produced by your partner. It is full of rich antibodies and nutrients to protect your baby.

- **Conception.** The process of becoming pregnant - when a sperm and egg join to form a single cell (alternative terms include "fertilisation", "impregnation", and "insemination").

- **Contraction.** Often strong and painful tightening of the uterus during labour that causes your partner's cervix to dilate, which helps push your baby through the birth canal.

- **Crowning.** The final stage of labour when your baby's head is visible at the vaginal opening (also known as the "ring of fire" because of the intensity of the process).

- **Delivery room.** A hospital area where babies are born (also called the "labour ward").

- **Dilation.** The process by which the cervix opens to allow your baby to pass through the birth canal. It's the first stage of labour.

- **Epidural.** A type of anaesthetic commonly used in labour where drugs are used to numb the lower half of the body to relieve pain during childbirth.

- **Estimated Date of Confinement (EDC).** The expected date of delivery for your pregnant partner (also known as the "estimated date of delivery" (EDD) or "due date").

- **Ferber Method.** A sleep training technique that helps your baby learn to fall asleep on their own (also known as "graduated extinction" or "graduated crying it out").

- **First trimester.** The first 12–14 weeks of pregnancy, from conception to the start of the second trimester.

- **Fontanelles.** The soft spots on your baby's head that allow its skull to compress during birth so it can pass through the birth canal.

- **Forceps.** A tong-shaped instrument placed around a baby's head to help it travel through the birth canal during childbirth.

- **Full term.** The normal duration of pregnancy (between 37 and 42 weeks gestation).

- **Gestational diabetes (GDM).** A condition that occurs during pregnancy when the body can't produce enough insulin to control blood sugar levels. This results in high blood sugar or hyperglycemia.

- **Gynaecologist.** A doctor who has undertaken specialist training in women's health.

- **Hypnobirthing.** A method of pain management that can be used during labour and childbirth.

- **Immunisation.** The process of receiving a vaccine, often by injection, to build immunity to certain bacteria or viruses (also known as a "vaccination").

- **Incontinence.** An inability to control your bladder or bowel movements.

- **Induction.** The process of stimulating labour to start artificially.

- **Jaundice.** A condition where your skin, the whites of your eyes and mucous membranes (like the inside of your nose and mouth) take on a yellowish tinge caused by an excess of a chemical called bilirubin in the blood.

- **Labour.** The process of a baby moving through the birth canal and out of the uterus (also called "childbirth").

- **Labour ward.** A hospital area where women give birth (also called the "delivery room or suite").

- **Lactation consultant.** A health professional who specialises in breastfeeding and chestfeeding. They can help with breastfeeding problems, provide education, and offer emotional support.

- **Maternal and child health nurse.** A trained nurse who specialises in managing the health of both mother and child throughout the reproductive and early developmental stages.

- **Meconium.** This is the first poo a newborn passes. Passing this before birth may be a sign of fetal distress.

- **Midwife.** A health professional specially trained to care for women during pregnancy, labour, birth and post-birth.

- **Morning sickness.** Nausea, vomiting, and aversion to certain foods and smells during pregnancy.

- **Mucus Plug.** A thick, gel-like collection of mucus that blocks the opening of the cervix to prevent bacteria from entering the uterus.

- **Neonatal period.** The first four weeks of a baby's life.

- **Neonatal Intensive Care Unit (NICU).** A specialised hospital ward where critically ill or premature newborn babies receive intensive medical care, including monitoring, life support, and specialised treatments.

- **Neonate.** A baby who is a few hours, days, or up to 4 weeks old (also known as "newborn).

- **Nursery.** A room in a hospital where babies are cared for.

- **Obstetrician.** A physician who specialises in delivering babies and caring for women during pregnancy and after birth.

- **Paediatrician.** A doctor with special training in preventing, diagnosing, and treating diseases and injuries in children.

- **Placenta.** A temporary organ that connects to the uterus wall and nourishes your baby through the umbilical cord.

- **Postnatal.** The period after giving birth (also known as "post-birth" and "postpartum').

- **Postnatal depression (PND).** A condition that affects some mothers in the days, weeks or months after giving birth (also known as "postpartum depression").

- **Preeclampsia.** A pregnancy complication that causes high blood pressure and protein in the urine. It can also cause damage to other organs.

- **Premature birth.** When a baby is born before 37 weeks of pregnancy (also known as "preterm birth").

- **Prenatal.** The time before birth or the period of pregnancy (also known as "antenatal" and "antepartum").

- **Second-stage labour.** The time from the complete dilation of the cervix to the birth of your baby.

- **Second trimester.** The middle period of pregnancy, usually lasting from weeks 13–27 (also called the "honeymoon period" because many of the unpleasant symptoms of early pregnancy subside).

- **Sleep regression.** A temporary period when a child's sleep patterns change, making it difficult for them to fall or stay asleep.

- **Spontaneous labour.** When labour begins naturally, without the use of drugs or other techniques.

- **Sudden Infant Death Syndrome (SIDS).** The sudden and unexplained death of an otherwise healthy baby, usually during sleep.

- **Transcutaneous Electrical Nerve Stimulation (TENS) machine.** Uses electrical impulses to relieve pain during labour.

- **Theatre.** A room in a hospital where surgical operations are performed.

- **Third-stage labour.** The time from the birth of the baby to the delivery of the placenta (also known as "afterbirth").

- **Third trimester.** The final stage of pregnancy, lasting from about 28 weeks to 40 weeks, or until birth.

- **Trimesters.** The three stages of pregnancy, each lasting about three months.

- **Ultrasound.** An imaging test that uses sound waves to create pictures of your baby inside the womb (also known as a "sonogram").

- **Umbilical cord.** The tube-like structure that connects the baby to the placenta during pregnancy, allowing nutrients and oxygen to be carried from the mother to her baby.

- **Uterus.** Where an unborn baby develops and grows (also known as "the womb").

- **Vacuum cap.** A suction cap that is sometimes used during birth to help pull the baby out of the birth canal (also known as a "ventouse" or "vacuum extractor").

- **Vaginal Birth After Caesarean (VBAC).** When a woman has a vaginal birth after having had one or more previous caesarean sections.

- **Viable pregnancy.** A pregnancy that is likely to continue to full term.

- **Water breaking.** When the protective sac of fluid around your baby breaks, allowing fluid to leak out (also known as rupture of the membranes).

Parenting Lingo

- **Attachment parenting (AP).** A style of parenting using genuine sensitivity, endless support, and love, forming a close bond believed to bring out the best in the child.

- **Au pair.** A young adult who lives with a host family and helps with childcare and housework.

- **Baby blues.** A temporary feeling of sadness after giving birth.

- **Baby brain.** A condition of impaired memory, concentration, or mental agility sometimes experienced by a woman during pregnancy or after giving birth.

- **Baby bump.** The round, enlarged abdomen of a pregnant woman.

- **Baby gym.** A play space for babies that includes a frame, a play mat, and hanging toys, and helps them develop their motor skills and hand-eye coordination.

- **Babymoon.** A relaxing or romantic holiday taken by parents-to-be before their baby is born.

- **Babyproofing.** Making your home safe for a baby by reducing or removing potential hazards.

- **Baby's first.** A special event or milestone for a baby.

- **Babywearing.** The practice of wearing or carrying a baby in a sling or another form of carrier.

- **Baby whipped.** Being completely controlled by your tiny, drooling baby.

- **Blowout.** When your baby poops so much that it explodes outside of his diaper and causes a giant, stinky mess.

- **Booger sucker.** A device that uses suction to remove mucus and fluid from your baby's nose (also known as a "nasal aspirator").

- **Boppy.** A C-shaped pillow commonly used to offer support when nursing or bottle feeding.

- **Bouncer.** A seat that gently rocks, bounces or vibrates to soothe your baby.

- **Breastfeeding.** The action of feeding your baby breast milk (also known as nursing).

- **Burp cloth.** A cloth used to catch spit-ups or burps from your baby.

- **Butt paste.** A diaper rash cream that helps protect your baby's skin from moisture and treat diaper skin irritations.

- **Co-sleeping.** When a parent and baby share a bed or sleep close together for easy breastfeeding, constant bonding, and a feeling of security (be aware of potential co-sleeping risks like accidental smothering and children falling off the bed).

- **Cot.** A baby's bed with high sides to keep them safe (also known as a crib).

- **Cry It Out (CIO).** Allowing your baby to cry until they fall asleep on their own.

- **Dad brain.** A term used to describe the changes in a man's brain after he becomes a father.

- **Doula.** A non-medical professional, usually a woman, who provides support during pregnancy, labour, and birth or after giving birth.

- **Dream feeding.** Nursing or bottle-feeding your baby at night without fully waking them up.

- **Dummy.** A nipple-shaped object for babies to suck on for comfort (also known as a "pacifier" or "binky").

- **Extended family involvement.** Involving relatives beyond the immediate nuclear family - grandparents, aunts, uncles, etc - in childcare. A common practice in many cultures.

- **Feeding cues.** Signs a baby gives when they are hungry.

- **Goo goo gaga.** Baby talk or cooing noises babies make before they learn to speak real words.

- **Grandparenting.** The act of a grandparent participating in the upbringing of their grandchild.

- **Helicopter parent.** An overbearing, over-focused parent who is overly involved and controlling in their child's life (also known as "cosseting parenting").

- **High chair.** A chair that allows your baby to sit at table height for meals.

- **Lawnmower parent.** A parent who "mows down" any obstacles to prevent their child from experiencing discomfort or disappointment (also known as "bulldoze parenting").

- **Layette.** A collection of clothing, bedding, and accessories for your newborn baby.

- **Lovey.** An overly loved stuffed animal or blanket that a child has grown attached to over time.

- **Me time.** Time spent relaxing on one's own instead of working or doing things for others.

- **Milk drunk.** When a baby looks blissfully sleepy after a good feeding.

- **Moses basket.** A smaller, portable bed for newborns (also known as a "bassinet").

- **Mombie.** A mother consumed by raising her children to the point of being sleep-deprived.

- **Mommy brain.** A term used to describe the forgetfulness and brain fog that some new mothers experience during pregnancy and after giving birth

- **Naptime.** The time of day when a baby takes a short period of sleep, usually in addition to their main nighttime sleep

- **Nappy.** A piece of towelling or other absorbent material wrapped around your baby's bottom and between its legs to absorb and retain wee and poo (what the British call a "diaper").

- **Onesie.** A soft, comfortable one-piece garment for infants and babies with snaps at the crotch for easy access to diaper changes (also known as a "baby grow suit").

- **Pee pee tee pee.** A cotton "tent" used to cover baby boy's penis and to prevent the parent from getting peed on during a diaper change, essentially acting as a "pee shield".

- **Playtime.** Time for a baby to explore, learn and develop through play.

- **Sleep like a baby.** Sleeping deeply and soundly.

- **Snuggle bug.** A baby who enjoys cuddling.

- **Stay-at-home mum (SAHM).** A mother who stays at home to raise her children.

- **Stay-at-home dad (SAHD).** A father who stays at home to raise his children.

- **Self-soothing.** The action of a young child ceasing to cry without being comforted, particularly when left to fall asleep on their own.

- **Sleep deprived.** Lacking enough sleep.

- **Sleep training.** Teaching a baby to sleep through the night.

- **Stroller.** A pushable chair on wheels for taking your baby on the go (also known as a "pram").

- **Tiger mum.** A very strict and demanding mother who pushes her child to succeed.

- **Tiny human.** A loving nickname for a baby.

- **Tired but wired.** A state of feeling exhausted and mentally alert at the same time.

- **Trying to Conceive (TTC).** Used to describe the process of attempting to get pregnant (also called "baby dancing").

- **Tummy Time.** Time spent by a baby lying on their stomach while awake, intended to help develop strength in the neck, arms, back, etc.

- **Washcloth.** Used to describe the process of attempting to get pregnant (also called a "facecloth", "flannel", or "washrag").

Developmental Milestones

- **Fine Motor Skills.** The precise movements of your child's hands, fingers, wrists, feet, and toes. They include picking up small objects, writing and drawing.

- **Gross Motor Skills.** The movements that use the body's large muscles to perform tasks. They include crawling, walking, running, and jumping.

- **Language Development.** The process by which your child learns to communicate and understand speech. It involves learning to speak, understanding others, and expressing their own thoughts and feelings.

- **Social-Emotional Development.** The process of learning to understand and express emotions and how to interact with others. It's the foundation for relationships and interactions in a child's life.

- **Cognitive Development.** The process by which your child learns, thinks, explores, and figures things out. This includes learning to respond to voices and facial expressions.

- **Physical Development.** The growth and change of your child's body, including muscles, bones, and other parts.

Feeding and Nutrition Vocab

- **Baby-led weaning (BLW).** A method of introducing solid food into a baby's diet by allowing them to feed themselves instead of being spoon-fed.

- **Breastfeeding.** The act of feeding breast milk to an infant.

- **Breast Milk.** Milk produced by a woman's body to feed her baby.

- **Cluster Feeding.** When a baby feeds more frequently than usual, often in the evening.

- **Donor Milk.** Breast milk donated by a mother and processed by a milk bank for use by another baby.

- **Expressed Breast Milk.** Breast milk that has been pumped and stored for later use.

- **Finger Foods.** Small pieces of food that are easy for babies to hold and eat.

- **Formula.** A specially treated milk powder that's mixed with water and given to babies in bottles.

- **Formula Feeding.** The practice of feeding a baby with infant formula instead of or in addition to breast milk.

- **Purée.** A very smooth, crushed or blended food that is often made from fruits, vegetables, meats, or whole grains. Purees are traditionally the first solid foods that babies eat.

- **Weaning.** Transitioning your baby from breast milk or formula to solid foods.

References

- *1 in 10 Dads Experience Postpartum Depression, Anxiety: How to Spot the Signs. (2021).* UT Southwestern Medical Center. https://utswmed.org/medblog/paternal-postpartum-depression/

- *6 Signs Your Baby is Hungry.* Strong4Life. (n.d.). https://www.strong4life.com/en/feeding-and-nutrition/hunger-and-fullness-cues/6-signs-your-baby-is-hungry#is-your-baby-hungry-here-are-6-signs

- *30 Heartfelt Ways to Thank Your Family Caregiver during National Family Caregiver Month.* (n.d.). Aidaly. https://aidaly.com/post/30-heartfelt-ways-to-thank-family-caregiver-during-national-family-caregiver-month

- *A to Z of Parenting Terms (Glossary of Terms).* (n.d.). Thisdadcan.co.uk. https://www.thisdadcan.co.uk/a-z-of-parenting-terms/

- *All About Skin-to-Skin Contact (Kangaroo Care).* (2024). Pampers. https://www.pampers.com/en-us/pregnancy/giving-birth/article/skin-to-skin-contact

- *Babies - Consumer Reports.* (2024). Consumer Reports. https://www.consumerreports.org/babies/

- *Dad's Guide to Pregnancy.* (2025). BabyCenter. https://www.babycentre.co.uk/pregnancy/dads

- **Barda, G., Mizrachi, Y., Borokchovich, I., Yair, L., Kertesz, D. P., & Dabby, R.** (2021). *The Effect of Pregnancy on Maternal Cognition.* Scientific Reports, 11(1), 12187. https://doi.org/10.1038/s41598-021-91504-9

- **Benedictus, L.** (n.d.). *The Father Hood - The Hood for Fathers.* The Father Hood. https://www.the-father-hood.com/article/fatherhood-can-steal-your-identity-heres-how-to-get-it-back/

- *Tummy Time for a Healthy Baby.* (n.d.). Safe to Sleep®. https://safetosleep.nichd.nih.gov/reduce-risk/tummy-time

- *Best Apps to Help Working Parents Juggle Work/Life Balance.* (2018). https://www.thriving-parents.com/blog/best-apps-to-help-working-parents-juggle-daily-tasks-and-work-life-balance

- **Bouchez, C.** (2005). *Pregnant Passions: Keep Intimacy Alive.* WebMD. https://www.webmd.com/women/features/intimacy-and-pregnancy

- **Buswell, G.** (2025). *Childcare Options for Families in the UK.* Expatica United Kingdom. https://www.expatica.com/uk/living/family/the-childcare-system-in-the-uk-106598/

- *Car Seats and Booster Seats.* (n.d.). NHTSA. https://www.nhtsa.gov/equipment/car-seats-and-booster-seats

- **Cherry, K. N.** (2024). *The 20 Best Developmental Toys for Your Baby and Toddler.* Pathfinder Health. https://www.pathfinder.health/post/developmental-toys

- **Collingwood, J.** (2016). *Teaching Your Baby Sign Language Can Benefit Both of You.* Psych Central. https://psychcentral.com/lib/teaching-your-baby-sign-language-can-benefit-both-of-you

- *Cross-Cultural Similarities and Differences in Parenting.* (n.d.). nih.gov. https://pmc.ncbi.nlm.nih.gov/articles/PMC8940605/

- DAD Support Group. (2024). Postpartum Support International (PSI). https://www.postpartum.net/group/dad-support-group/

- **Degges-White, S., PhD.** (2023). *10 Steps to Effective Couples Communication | How can you make discussions with your partner more productive?* Psychology Today. https://www.psychologytoday.com/us/blog/lifetime-connections/201605/10-steps-to-effective-couples-communication

- **Dennis, J. G.** (2024). *Writing a Family Mission Statement. Focus on the Family.* https://www.focusonthefamily.com/parenting/writing-a-family-mission-statement/

- **Downs, M., MPH.** (2009). *An Expectant Dad's Guide to Pregnancy.* WebMD. https://www.webmd.com/baby/features/an-expectant-dads-guide-to-pregnancy

- *Education in the UK vs US: Full Comparison (2024).* (2024). Kings Education. https://www.kingseducation.com/kings-life/education-in-uk-vs-us

- **Ellingwood, J.** (2024). *10 Healthy Family Communication Skills and How to Implement Them.* Anchor Light Therapy. https://anchorlighttherapy.com/family-communication/

- **Emery, L., Libera, A., Lehman, E., & Levi, B. H.** (2024). *Humor in Parenting: Does it Have a Role?* PLoS ONE, 19(7), e0306311. https://doi.org/10.1371/journal.pone.0306311

- *Fetal Development | Week-by-Week Stages of Pregnancy.* (2024). Cleveland Clinic. https://my.clevelandclinic.org/health/articles/7247-fetal-development-stages-of-growth

- *Fourth Trimester.* (n.d.). the Bump. https://www.thebump.com/topics/fourth-trimester

- **Gordon, S.** (2024). *What are the Five Love Languages?* Verywell Mind. https://www.verywellmind.com/can-the-five-love-languages-help-your-relationship-4783538

- **Gouw, T.** (2020). *8 Apps Every New Dad Needs on His Phone.* Medium. https://medium.com/@punttim/7-apps-every-new-dad-needs-on-his-phone-b0b9fbaa7fad

- **Gritters, J.** (2025). *The 4 Best Baby Carriers, Tested and Approved by Parents and Kids.* Forbes. https://www.forbes.com/sites/forbes-personal-shopper/article/best-baby-carriers/

- **Hartshorn, J.** (2024). *Must-Have Baby Essentials for Your Registry.* Parents. https://www.parents.com/baby/gear/registries-buying-guides/baby-shopping-guide/

- *Helping Babies Sleep Safely.* (2024). Reproductive Health. https://www.cdc.gov/reproductive-health/features/babies-sleep.html

- **Hoffman, J.** (2023). *The Ultimate Rookie Dad Guide to Newborns.* Todaysparent.com. https://www.todaysparent.com/baby/newborn-care/a-rookie-dads-guide-to-newborns/

- **Holcombe, M.** (2024). *Even if Your Kids Roll Their Eyes, Keep Making Jokes, research says.* CNN. https://www.cnn.com/2024/07/18/health/humor-parenting-wellness/index.html

- **Hope, C.** (2020). *Uninsured and Unemployed? Medicaid and CHIP Provide Lifelines to Families in Need.* Center for Children and Families. https://ccf.georgetown.edu/2020/04/21/what-help-is-available-for-uninsured-during-covid-19-pandemic/

- How Dads Can Support Their Breastfeeding Partner. (n.d.). https://wicbreastfeeding.fns.usda.gov/how-dads-can-support-their-breastfeeding-partner

- **Immaculate, A.** (2024). *Childproofing Your Home.* Parents Africa. https://parentsafrica.com/childproofing-your-home/

- **Kagan, J.** (2024). *529 Plan: What it is, How it Works, Pros and Cons.* Investopedia. https://www.investopedia.com/terms/1/529plan.asp

- **Katie.** (2025). *10 Best Books for First-Time Dads.* Peacock Parent. https://peacockparent.com/10-best-books-for-first-time-dads/

- **Kawashima, C.** (2024). *6 Financial Planning Tips for New Parents.* Schwab Brokerage. https://www.schwab.com/learn/story/6-financial-planning-tips-new-parents

- **Keefe, J.** (2023). *Baby Checklist.* MoneySavingExpert.com. https://www.moneysavingexpert.com/family/baby-checklist/

- **Korolkovaite, I.** (2017). *Parents are Posting Their Most Epic Fails, and it's Hilarious.* Bored Panda. https://www.boredpanda.com/funny-parenting-fails/

- **LaBracio, J., CPST.** (2024). *Ultimate Hospital Bag Checklist for Mom and baby.* Babylist. https://www.babylist.com/hello-baby/what-to-pack-in-your-hospital-bag

- *Laughter Therapy: A Humor-Induced Hormonal Intervention to Reduce Stress and Anxiety.* (2021). nih.gov. https://pmc.ncbi.nlm.nih.gov/articles/PMC8496883/

- *Learn First Aid for Babies and Children.* (n.d.). British Red Cross. https://www.redcross.org.uk/first-aid/learn-first-aid-for-babies-and-children

- **Lemire, S.** (2025). *275 Best Dad Jokes to Tickle Everyone's Funny Bone.* TODAY.com. https://www.today.com/life/dad-jokes-rcna27325

- **Links, A. R., Callon, W., Wasserman, C., Walsh, J., Beach, M. C., & Boss, E. F.** (2019). *Surgeon Use of Medical Jargon with Parents in the Outpatient Setting.* Patient Education and Counselling. https://doi.org/10.1016/j.pec.2019.02.002

- **McConnell, L.** (2022). *8 (Realistic) Ways Working Dads Can Achieve Work-Life Balance.* Ivy Exec. https://ivyexec.com/career-advice/2022/8-realistic-ways-working-dads-can-achieve-work-life-balance

- **Miles, K.** (2024). *Benefits of Skin-to-Skin Contact with Your Newborn.* BabyCenter. https://www.babycenter.com/baby/newborn-baby/benefits-of-skin-to-skin-contact-with-your-newborn_20005036

- **Mohammed, S., Afaya, A., & Abukari, A. S.** (2023). *Reading, Singing, and Storytelling: The Impact of Caregiver-Child Interaction and Child Access to Books and Preschool on Early Childhood Development in Ghana.* Scientific Reports. https://doi.org/10.1038/s41598-023-38439-5

- *Morning Sickness - Diagnosis and Treatment.* (n.d.). Mayo Clinic. https://www.mayoclinic.org/diseases-conditions/morning-sickness/diagnosis-treatment/drc-20375260

- *National Breastfeeding Month.* (2022). Redline Specialty Pharmacy. https://www.redlinepharmacy.com/national-breastfeeding-month/

- *New Dads & Partners: How Your Involvement Matters.* (2024). HealthyChildren.org. https://www.healthychildren.org/English/ages-stages/baby/Pages/A-Special-Message-to-Fathers.aspx

- **Ninivaggi, F. J., M. D.** (2023). *How the Role of Being a Dad is Changing.* Psychology Today. https://www.psychologytoday.com/us/blog/envy-this/202305/fatherhood-in-2023

- *Our Favorite Baby-Proofing Tools.* (2019). The New York Times. https://www.nytimes.com/wirecutter/reviews/our-favorite-baby-proofing-tools/

- *Paid Parental Leave: Big Differences for Mothers and Fathers.* (2023). OECD statistics. https://oecdstatistics.blog/2023/01/12/paid-parental-leave-big-differences-for-mothers-and-fathers/

- **Parlakian, R.** (2023). *Play Activities for Birth to 12 months.* Zero to Three.

https://www.zerotothree.org/resource/play-activities-for-birth-to-12-months/

- *Pregnancy.* (2025). NHS. https://www.nhs.uk/pregnancy/

- *Pregnancy Complications.* (2024). Maternal Infant Health. https://www.cdc.gov/maternal-infant-health/pregnancy-complications/index.html

- *Pregnancy: Physical Changes After Delivery.* (2025). Cleveland Clinic. https://my.clevelandclinic.org/health/articles/9682-pregnancy-physical-changes-after-delivery

- **Reid, S.** (2024). *Empathy: How to Feel and Respond to the Emotions of Others.* HelpGuide.org. https://www.helpguide.org/relationships/communication/empathy

- *Relationships After Having a Baby.* (2023). NHS. https://www.nhs.uk/conditions/baby/support-and-services/relationships-after-having-a-baby/

- **Russell, A.** (2023). *28 Fun and Meaningful Family Traditions to Treasure Forever.* Remento. https://www.remento.co/journal/fun-and-meaningful-family-traditions-to-treasure-forever

- **Sachs, L., & Constantine, A.** (2023). *7 Best Diapers for Babies, According to Product Experts and Parents.* Good Housekeeping. https://www.goodhousekeeping.com/childrens-products/diaper-reviews/g19502261/best-diapers/

- **Spurrier, J., MD.** (2025). *Best Baby Gear of 2025: Top 88 Products.* GearLab. https://www.babygearlab.com/topics/baby-and-kids/best-baby-gear

- **Staff, B.** (2023). *Acronyms, Abbreviations, and Emoticons!* BabyCenter. https://www.babycenter.com/community-help-abbreviations

- *Stages of Labor and Birth: Baby, it's time!* (n.d.). Mayo Clinic. https://www.mayoclinic.org/healthy-lifestyle/labor-and-delivery/in-depth/stages-of-labor/art-20046545

- **Tam, S.** (2023). *Activities for Bonding and Learning from Birth to 12 months.* Zero to Three. https://www.zerotothree.org/resource/activities-for-bonding-and-learning-from-birth-to-12-months/

- **Team, B.** (2023). *How to Create the Perfect Sleep Sanctuary for Your Little*

- *One*. Natemia. https://natemia.com/blogs/natemia-blog/how-to-create-the-perfect-sleep-sanctuary-for-your-little-one

- *The Birth Plan – Dad's Adventure*. (n.d.). https://dadsadventure.com/the-birth-plan/

- *The Essential Guide for New Dads | Support Guide for new Dads*. (2025). DadPad. https://thedadpad.co.uk/

- *The Importance of Empathy in Relationships*. (2022). Array Behavioral Care. https://arraybc.com/the-importance-of-empathy-in-relationships

- *The New Parent's Survival Guide: Surviving your Baby's First Week*. (2020). Family Compassion. https://www.family-compassion.org/post/the-new-parent-s-survival-guide-surviving-your-baby-s-first-week

- **Villano, M.** (2024). *When Dad Struggles After the Baby Arrives*. Seleni Institute. https://seleni.org/advice-support/2018/3/12/when-dad-struggles-after-the-baby-arrives

- **Wall, C.** (2024). *Eco-Chic: A Guide to Stylish, Safe, and Sustainable Baby Products for Your Registry*. Lalo. https://www.meetlalo.com/blogs/news/eco-chic-a-guide-to-stylish-safe-and-sustainable-baby-products-for-your-registry?srsltid=AfmBOooX7bbVY6nYbCYKDdLWNgmnNcGx2Q4mL88UZAoUGuL3q9SbQT8D

- *Important Milestones: Your Child By One Year* (2024). Centers for Disease Control and Prevention. https://www.cdc.gov/ncbddd/actearly/milestones/milestones-1yr.html

- *When Can a Child Stop Using a Booster Seat?* (2023). Happy Family Blog. https://happyfamilyblog.com/when-can-a-child-stop-using-a-booster-seat/

- *Where to Find Your Parenting Mentor*. (2021). The ONE Thing. https://the1thing.com/where-to-find-your-parenting-mentor/

- *Work Out Your Baby Budget*. (n.d.). Money Helper. https://www.moneyhelper.org.uk/en/family-and-care/becoming-a-parent/baby-costs-calculator

- **Zalewski, P.** (2022). *A Definitive Checklist for New Dads (check these boxes, dads-to-be!)*. Fathercraft.com. https://fathercraft.com/checklist-for-new-dads/?srsltid=AfmBOooGs_AoiR5EtcZnRLNFtCRF3-g2gOhIZe3ZKCe7OSTDJZoG5jeB

Keep the Dadhood Spirit Alive

Now that you've got the tips and tools to tackle dadhood like a pro, it's time to pay it forward. Share what you've learned and show other dads where they can find the same advice and support.

By leaving your honest opinion of this book on Amazon, you'll help another dad - or dad-to-be - find the guidance they're searching for, and pass on the passion for navigating dadhood with confidence (and maybe a laugh or two).

Thank you for helping to keep the dadhood spirit alive, one shared word at a time. Together, we're making the journey a little easier and a lot more meaningful for every dad out there.

Simply scan the QR code to leave your review on Amazon.

Still your biggest fan,

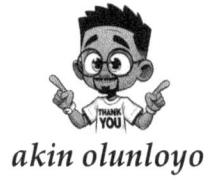

akin olunloyo

We hope you enjoyed this Syncterface Media book.
If you'd like to find out more about Syncterface Media,
please contact:

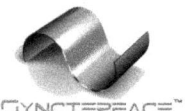

info@syncterfacemedia.com
www.syncterfacemedia.com

www.ingramcontent.com/pod-product-compliance
Lightning Source LLC
Chambersburg PA
CBHW061230070526
44584CB00030B/4055